midlife newlife

SO-ATE-254

BARNES
& NOBLE
BOOKS

NEW YORK

renewal, rejuvenation & new direction

Judith Wills

special photography by **Liz McAulay**

midlife
new life

To Tony, the inspiration for much, both in this book and in my life

This edition published by Barnes & Noble, Inc., by arrangement with Quadrille Publishing Ltd.

2005 Barnes & Noble Books

M 10 9 8 7 6 5 4 3 2 1

Editorial Director **Jane O'Shea**
Editor & Project Manager **Lewis Esson**
Art Director **Mary Evans**
Production **Jane Rogers**
Illustration **Bridget Bodoano**
Photography **Liz McAulay**
Styling **Claire Roberts**
Make-up **Dottie Monaghan** and **James McMahon**

Text © Judith Wills 2004
Photography © see page 237
Design & layout © Quadrille Publishing Ltd 2004

The rights of Judith Wills to be identified as the Author of this Work have been asserted by her in accordance with the Copyright, Designs and Patents Act 1988.

All rights reserved. No part of this book may be reproduced, stored in a retrieval system or transmitted in any form or by any means, electronic, electrostatic, magnetic tape, mechanical, photocopying, recording or otherwise, without the prior permission in writing of the publisher.

Cataloguing in Publication Data: a catalogue record for this book is available from the British Library

ISBN 0-7607-7483-8

Printed in China

introduction

Midlife...You... Can you believe it? Well—DID you ever really think you'd reach half a century or so? I certainly didn't—but I got there, somehow!

This book aims to prove that being "middle aged" is no reason for depression and might even be a cause for celebration—the start of your new life. I have tried hard not to offer false hope of a return to the physical fitness or shape of youth, or to peddle miracle cures to keep you alive, fertile, or wrinkle-free to 150. However, I firmly believe—and know—that everything you don't like about yourself can be improved, all the baggage that comes with no longer being 20 can be a blessing not a deadweight, and that at any time from your late forties through to your sixties you can, if you choose, begin the most fulfilling—even exciting—decades of your life.

As we are all living longer than ever before, you've got at least forty or fifty years of good (in its best sense) living ahead, with a bit of luck. And we "baby boomers" are lucky in that many of us do have better health, healthier finances, and more opportunities than any other generation before us.

In *Midlife, New Life*, I have set out to make the most of this good fortune. I wanted to document all that can realistically be achieved once we are no longer in the state known as youth; to encourage you to try what is documented and, most importantly, to tell the truth. From food to physical fitness, from health to libido and emotions, if you need guidance and motivation, I hope you will find them here.

Judith Wills

January 2004

fuel for your newlife

Food is fundamental to our total well-being, health, and existence. What we eat IS at least some of what we are—which is why I describe food as "fuel."

Although there are other influences on how good you feel, how long you live, and how healthy you are, the right fuel is certainly one of the most important factors in defining how well you function.

In Chapter 1, we will be looking at all the ways in which the right body fuel is empowering. In midlife, a good diet is especially relevant. It may be time to alter long-standing food habits that aren't serving you well. Time to prime your body for the inevitable changes of the years ahead.

Certainly, the ideas that we discuss here should enhance your life, not hamper it. Good food and drink are not only priorities—but pleasures. Don't miss out.

what do you eat? Your diet makes a difference to your life in so many ways.

How do you feel today? How do you feel this very minute? How will you feel next week, next year—or in ten or twenty years' time? Believe it or not, immediate, short-term, and long-term health and well-being are, to a surprising degree, governed by what you eat and drink. (And, of course, by what you don't.)

A good diet—together with adequate exercise—is among the most important markers of a healthy and long life. Yet only in recent years has this been recognized by "officialdom," from the World Health Organization through national government health departments, and finally the message is being accepted by every one of us: we are what we eat.

Knowing the message and finding the motivation to act on it are different matters. In this section, Fuel for Your New Life, we offer that motivation by looking in detail at how a good diet can effect sometimes almost miraculous improvements in so many areas of our well-being.

We look at how the physical and mental aging process is affected by food, and at how the major diseases of the twenty-first century—such as cancers, heart disease, diabetes, high blood pressure, and arthritis—can be kept at bay. Of course, we are all different, and you will find out how to get an optimum diet whether you are 40, 50, or 60. Find out the truth about antioxidants and check out how many of the Top 20 Antiaging Foods appear regularly in your diet. Eat with an eye on your looks, because skin, hair, eyes, and "sparkle" can all improve.

Few people feel their best when they are carrying extra pounds that weren't there a decade ago. Find out the truth about middle-age spread and dieting at 40-plus, and get practical help on dealing with cellulite and hard-to-shift fat, lumps, and bumps.

Does detoxing really work? IS there actually such a thing? We look at the facts behind all the detox myths and help you decide whether a detox plan could work for you. Our effective but gentle program gives you the benefits of detoxing without any unwanted side effects.

Around the age of 50, diet becomes a major factor for many women in beating the negative symptoms of the menopause, and we provide everything you need to know—from eating to help minimize hot flashes and headaches to increasing energy and libido.

There really are "brain foods" that can help you retain your powers of concentration, memory, and sharpness. We look at helping you to optimum brain power through not only eating the right foods and avoiding the wrong ones, but by eating the right foods at the right times.

This chapter offers a variety of eating plans from which you can select to suit your own needs. Whichever plan you do choose, enjoyment of your menus should be a top priority. So here is a special plea—take time to find real pleasure in your menu planning and food shopping, even if you are only preparing meals for yourself. Buy the best-quality foods you can, enjoy cooking, and savor every mouthful. For busy midlifers who have spent many years too busy to cook or too busy making meals for others to really enjoy food—now is the time to start.

food and **antiaging**

The quality and length of your life, and your appearance and health as you age, can, to a large extent, be governed by you—and the decisions you make about what to eat and drink will form a very important part of the picture. Happily, it is never too late to start making those decisions the right ones.

Research shows that up to 75 percent of the aging process is not genetic. In other words, how well you age is largely under your own control. Diet is an important component of this self-help antiaging process. The typical signs of aging—the onset of conditions like cancer, heart disease, or diabetes, decline in general health and vitality, the appearance of wrinkles, and changes in hair and skin texture—can be kept at bay by a good diet or exacerbated by a poor one.

What you eat can not only slow down the speed at which you age, but to a certain extent can also turn back the clock —actually helping you to look and feel younger. Although this is not usually a fast process, you should notice certain improvements, such as increased energy or better skin, within as little as a week. Improvements in health—for example, a reduction in joint pain, tiredness, or blood pressure—can take from weeks to months.

First we look at eating right from early midlife, around forty, through the fifties, and into your sixties. Knowing what to eat and what not to eat—and choosing the right foods for energy—is important whatever your age, but the optimum mix of foods can vary according to your current decade.

Most people have heard the words "antioxidants" and "phytochemicals," but many are unsure of how these help, or even what they are. We help you make sense of these potent plant components and list the Top 20 Antiaging Foods.

Later in the chapter you will find specific advice for keeping your looks—skin, eyes, hair, and so on—in good condition, and finally there is a choice of diet plans, one of which will be your own blueprint for antiaging.

eat for your age

around 40

The early 40s are a hectic few years for most people—with children still at home, a career still in need of complete focus, personal relationships to maintain. Juggling time is an every-day necessity—and when life is that busy, healthy eating might be the last thing on your mind.

However, a few simple dietary tips can help you feel much better, give you more energy, help you sleep better, and beat the small, but often long-term, symptoms of ill health that can result from stress, or simply the beginnings of getting older.

how to eat
A speedy but nourishing breakfast is vital every day, to help your brain and body work better. Research shows that people who skip breakfast perform more poorly in the morning, they lack concentration, and they can feel dizzy due to low blood sugar.

Breakfast should include some complex carbs, such as whole-wheat bread or a whole-grain cereal, some protein, such as an egg, yogurt, or milk, a little fat (present in many protein foods and also in butter or spreads), and nuts and seeds—excellent foods in their own right (see the Top 20 Antiaging Foods, pages 20–3). The Diet Plan for Your 40s (see page 28) includes suggestions for quick-and-easy breakfasts of this type.

Lunch should be reasonably low in carbohydrate and high in protein, as research shows that this will produce the best afternoon performance—too much carb will slow you down and can make you feel drowsy. Thus a chicken salad or fish and vegetables is better than two sandwiches or a plate of pasta. Again, you will find quick lunch ideas in the diet plans.

Around 4:30 or 5 p.m. you should get a small snack to restore your energy—an apple and a small piece of cheese, a pot of yogurt, or some fresh nuts are ideal energy foods that will keep your blood sugar level constant while you travel home from work, deal with children's meals, or work late.

Try to have your evening meal no later than 7:30 p.m. and organize your evenings so that time after 7 p.m. is all for you. Cooking a simple meal and savoring it should help you to relax and unwind. Include plenty of the Top 20 Antiaging Foods and make this meal higher in carbs than lunch. This will help you to wind your brain down toward bedtime.

Drinks Have at least 6 to 8 glasses of water or the equivalent each day to keep yourself hydrated properly. See Food and Detox (pages 48–53) and Food for Your Looks (pages 24–31).

eating for health
A general healthy diet—high in fresh fruits and veggies, grains, lean protein, nuts, seeds, and legumes—is recommended in the 40s as for any age, but pay particular attention to foods that provide you with sustained energy (see the Glycemic Index, page 38) and most meet your particular health needs. Check the box on the left for food tips for health problems typical at this age.

treats to savor
Don't feel you have to give up all your favorite edible treats or drinks to get your healthy diet. A glass or two of good-quality wine can be an excellent idea, too—but leave it at one or two glasses for optimum health and well-being benefits. (See the feature on alcohol and drugs in Well-being for Your New Life, pages 196–7.) In moderation, beer is an excellent drink in the evening, as hops are a sedative. Choose organic wine or beer to minimize the chance of a hangover and unwanted residues.

Chocolate can be very good for you because of its high antioxidant content—choose semisweet chocolate as it is highest in the beneficial cocoa solids. Tea and coffee are also rich in antioxidants and other plant chemicals that help protect against heart disease, while moderate amounts of coffee can increase alertness and concentration. Avoid caffeine-rich drinks with meals as it reduces absorption of vital minerals, like calcium and iron, and limit coffee intake to 4 cups a day.

If you suffer from ... **ibs** ... **try** honey, fresh herbs, fish, fruit, vegetables.

If you suffer from ... **headaches and migraine** ... **try** avoiding caffeine, hard cheese, alcohol – **and drink 6–8 glasses of water a day.**

If you suffer from ... **stress**... **try** milk, turkey, camomile tea, chocolate, complex carbs.

If you suffer from ... **pms** ... **try** avoiding caffeine, alcohol and simple carbohydrates, and drink plenty of fluids. **Eat foods rich in vitamin B, such as whole grains.**

foods to avoid

sugar The theory that sugar gives you energy is faulty—sugar contains calories, which are converted to energy in the body, but all food contains calories. Sugary items can give you a quick energy fix, but if you want sustaining energy to last for several hours, they are best avoided. They cause your blood sugar levels to rise quickly and then, as insulin floods the system to cope with this sugar, you can feel weak, light-headed, or tired.

This effect is heightened for women before a period. Avoid snacking on sugary foods alone (and this includes fruit) when you feel hungry and/or tired as you will simply compound the problem. Instead, go for the snacks mentioned in How to Eat on the left, or a small piece of wholemeal pita with hummus, or a tub of natural fromage blanc, or low-fat cottage cheese. Such snacks are low on the Glycemic Index, which measures how quickly food is absorbed into the bloodstream, and will keep you feeling energetic for longer, as well as keeping hunger at bay. Many simple carbohydrates, such as white bread, have a similar effect to sugar in the body. (See Food and Weight, pages 36–47 for more information on the Glycemic Index.)

alcohol during the day Most alcoholic drinks (even dry wine) contain a lot of sugar and have a similar effect on your blood sugar levels as sugary foods and refined carbohydrates. Avoid drinking alcohol during the day and stick to drinking a little with a meal in the evenings. Women who suffer PMS should avoid alcohol altogether in the week before a period, as research shows that intake exacerbates symptoms.

high caffeine intake While a small amount of caffeine spread out regularly is fine, excessive intake of high-caffeine beverages, such as brewed coffee or so-called "energy drinks," is not a good idea. These can place a strain on the adrenal system and can leave you feeling wiped out and jittery at the same time.

around 50

Eating preferences and habits can be entrenched by the age of 50, but not difficult to change if the need is there—and, as we get older, it is more important than ever to eat the foods that will help maintain health and ward off the signs of aging.

For women, healthy diet and weight maintenance can minimize the less desirable effects of the menopause, including hot flashes and tiredness. For more, see Food and Weight (pages 36–47) and Food for the Menopause (pages 54–9).

Although peak bone strength is built in youth, much can be done to help maintain bone density and thus reduce your chances of getting problems related to osteoporosis as you get older (see the box below). Osteoporosis is not only potentially life-threatening, highly debilitating, and the cause of most fractures in older people, but also unsightly, causing body shrinkage and postural changes—such as an exaggerated stoop that can add years to your real age.

At this time, much can also be done to help prevent the major killer diseases of later middle age and old age—cardiovascular disease and cancer. (See also Well-Being for Your New Life, page 168.)

bone builders

- Diet high in calcium (dairy produce, green leafy vegetables)
- Diet high in essential fatty acids (omega-3s and omega-6s)
- Weight-bearing exercise
- Diet high in fruit, vegetables
- Diet high in magnesium (nuts, seeds, whole grains) and vitamin E (plant oils, nuts, seeds)

bone robbers

- Diet high in animal protein
- Diet high in salt and the phosphates found in fizzy drinks and many processed foods
- Excessive consumption of alcohol and caffeine, and smoking
- Maintaining too low a body weight over time

do

● Eat up to 9 portions of fruit and vegetables a day. The latest information from the National Cancer Institute says that perhaps the recognized advice to eat 5 portions a day is, in fact, too low. Men should eat 9 and women 7. See Top 20 Antiaging Foods, pages 20–23, for the type of fruits and vegetables that can be particularly beneficial.

● Eat plenty of whole-grain foods. As well as helping to prevent certain cancers and reduce the risk of heart disease, they are also rich in nutrients and improve digestive efficiency.

● Eat legumes—for example soybeans, chickpeas, and lentils. The US government allows manufacturers of soy foods to make the claim that regular soy intake can help reduce high LDL blood cholesterol (the bad type), and all legumes are high in soluble fiber.

● Eat oily fish. Oily fish, such as salmon, herring, or mackerel, can help to prevent blood clots, heart disease, cancers, and arthritic pain.

● Eat garlic and onions—they contain a variety of compounds which both help to protect your circulatory health and can protect against cancer.

don't

● Eat too much high-fat animal food, such as shoulder of lamb, fatty cuts of beef, cheddar or Stilton cheese, or cream cheese, cream, or butter.

● Eat too many foods containing high levels of trans fats—fats that have been commercially hardened for use in mass-market products, such as margarines, cookies, cakes, pastries, and pies. These fats, also called hydrogenated fats, appear to be even worse for heart and circulatory health than natural saturated fats.

● Eat too many calories—being obese is a strain on the heart and obesity is also linked with increased risk of some cancers.

Maintaining a reasonable weight will also help to prevent the onset of insulin resistance, a precursor of diabetes and type-2 diabetes itself. Although it is often said that insulin resistance (when the body has to cope with too much sugar in the blood and its ability to produce sufficient insulin is blunted) is directly due to high sugar intake, that is, in fact, only partly true—a high intake of calories of any type over time (a surplus of which converts to glucose in the blood) is more likely to be the cause. If you eat moderate portions—think "little and often"—and get plenty of exercise, you are much less likely to suffer from either of these conditions.

around 60

From early middle age your calorie needs decline steadily, so monitor portion sizes carefully to make sure you don't put on too much weight, which can be very aging and can make you lethargic.

Research shows older people tend to crave sweet foods more than younger people, so try to satisfy your craving with natural foods, such as fresh or dried fruits, rather than with a lot of cakes, cookies, or candy. Choose top-quality honey rather than sugar, as it has healing properties. Try to keep your intake of salt reasonably low—high blood pressure is very common as you get older, and sodium intake can raise blood pressure in susceptible people.

As liver function and digestion may become sluggish, many people feel happier eating smaller meals more frequently, so 2 mini-meals, 2 snacks and 1 small main meal can be ideal. Alcohol tolerance can also decline—but one glass a day is still good news for heart health.

A diet high in antioxidant vitamins, minerals, and plant chemicals (see overleaf) will help protect you from disease and beat the signs of aging. With a healthy diet you shouldn't need food supplements—however, coenzyme Q10 can help maintain gum health and perhaps prevent the need for you ever to have false teeth! Fish oil supplements are an easy way to get your daily omega-3 oils with all their benefits (see Top 20 Antiaging Foods, pages 20–23).

Pain from arthritis and rheumatism can be minimized by eating ginger, chilies, and fish oils, and the risk of stroke can be halved with a diet high in potassium (bananas and onions, for example) and oily fish. Keep Alzheimer's and Parkinson's disease at bay with a diet rich in oily fish (again!), nuts, seeds, and olive oil, and maintain your eyesight by eating regular portions of carrots, mangoes, and dark green vegetables.

A generally healthy diet, containing plenty of antioxidant foods, is also the best way to maintain your immune system in good order and help keep colds and flu at bay.

know your nutrients
During midlife it is vital you get the optimum amount of all the "micronutrients" your body needs for good health and good functioning. Here we look at those nutrients, all needed in small but very important quantities, that can make all the difference to your health and well-being and how your body will age— and in the panel opposite we explain antioxidants and their vital role in holding back the aging process.

what are micronutrients?
They are vitamins, minerals, and phytochemicals (plant chemicals), and within this group I have also included essential fatty acids (special fats needed in small quantities, with a range of health benefits and antiaging qualities).

Vitamins are organic substances that are essential for a variety of roles in the body. The water-soluble vitamins are the B group (B_2, B_3, B_6, B_{12} and folate) and C, and these should be eaten every day, because they cannot be stored in the body. The fat-soluble vitamins, which the body can store, are vitamins A, D, E, and K.

Each vitamin has a different part to play in health, maintenance, and well-being, and the amount and balance that we need depend, among other things, upon our age. Some vitamins, such as C and beta-carotene (sometimes called pro-vitamin A, because the body can convert it into vitamin A) are also antioxidants (see opposite).

Vitamins B group and C are easily destroyed by storage, light, and heat, so foods containing these vitamins should be bought fresh, stored carefully, and given the minimum of cooking.

All vitamins are best consumed as a natural part of food, as researchers believe they can work synergistically with other compounds within foods. Supplements, however, can be useful on some occasions, (See Chapter 4 on well-being.)

minerals
are inorganic substances, fifteen of which are essential in the human diet, either to build and maintain structure (such as calcium and magnesium), or to balance body fluids (such as sodium and potassium), or to regulate body functions (such as iron and calcium). Some of these are occasionally, or even quite commonly, in short supply in the diet, and poor diet and lifestyle factors can hinder their absorption or increase their excretion. (This also applies to vitamins.)

The best way to guarantee an adequate intake and absorption of vitamins and minerals is to eat a balanced, healthy diet containing a wide variety of meat, fish, poultry, eggs, dairy produce, legumes, whole grains, nuts, seeds, fruit, and vegetables, and to lead a healthy lifestyle, avoiding excesses of alcohol, smoking, drugs, stress, and so on. Different sections and features in this book will refer to various mineral and vitamin needs for different problems and occasions.

essential fatty acids
The essential fatty acids (EFAs, otherwise known as "long-chain fatty acids") are part of the polyunsaturated family of fats. They are linoleic acid (the "parent" fat of the omega-6 group) and alphalinolenic acid (the "parent" fat of the omega-3 group). Approximately 2g a day of both of these are needed for good health.

While the modern diet tends to favor the linoleic acid/omega-6 fats (found in many plant oils, such as sunflower, safflower, corn, and sesame oil, and many modern processed foods), we might not get enough of the alphalinolenic acid/omega-3 group, as they are found mainly in oily fish and in smaller amounts in dark leafy greens, flax seeds, canold oil, and some nuts and seeds.

The correct balance and amount of these essential fats is linked with protection from heart disease, stroke, cancers, arthritis, immune system deficiencies, brain health, skin health, and much more. More on the EFAs appears in Chapter 4 on Well-Being for Your New Life.

making sense of antioxidants

Oxidation is a chemical reaction that occurs all the time in the human body when human cells convert oxygen and nutrients into energy. Oxidation can be seen in action when metal turns rusty. This oxidation in the body produces particles called "free radicals," natural by-products of everyday living.

However, when we age or are under stress or other negative lifestyle factors (for example, pollution, smoking, drinking, illness), free-radical production is increased and it is thought the physical signs of aging, as well as the diseases of old age, such as coronary heart disease (CHD) and cancers, are directly related to DNA damage caused by oxidation.

Certain substances in what we eat and drink can counteract oxidation and are, therefore, called antioxidants. Some vitamins and minerals, as well as a huge range of compounds in plants, have strong antioxidant properties. Scientists are now discovering that different types of antioxidants have different effects—for example, the compound in the spice turmeric called curcumin might be especially good at helping to prevent memory loss and Alzheimer's, while compounds called flavonoids, found in apples, onions, and wine, are particularly good at giving protection to the heart, and glucosinolates, found in leafy greens, broccoli, and cauliflower, can help to prevent cancers.

Some manufacturers have produced food-supplement capsules containing particular antioxidants, but it is not yet certain that these supplements are as potent as the "real thing"—proper food.

phytochemicals These are chemicals or compounds found in the plant foods that we eat (phyto = plant), which until recent years received little scientific attention but are now known to have important roles in health, antiaging, and disease prevention. Many of these phytochemicals are antioxidants (see above), while others can act as natural hormone balancers, anti-inflammatories, painkillers, antibiotics, and so on.

Fruits and vegetables are the main sources of phytochemicals in the diet, but whole grains, wine, beers, and honey also contain beneficial plant compounds. So far, about 12,000 different chemicals have been found by scientists, but new ones are being discovered all the time. A varied healthy diet including plenty of fresh produce is the simplest and best way to guarantee you get a good range of these powerful health allies.

top 20 antiaging foods

The right foods can not only hold off the aging process—helping you to look and feel younger—but can also protect you from many of the diseases and problems of old age.

These twenty foods are among the most important you should eat on a regular basis.

apples

Apples are rich in two phytochemicals (plant compounds) called catechins and quercetin. Both these help to prevent stroke, heart disease, and cancer. Quercetin has also been shown to improve the firmness of collagen, a component of skin that helps it to keep its elasticity and youthful appearance. Apples are also rich in the soluble fiber pectin, which helps to lower blood cholesterol. Lastly, the flesh of apples contains the mineral boron, which helps to prevent loss of calcium from the body and therefore helps prevent osteoporosis.

avocados

Avocados contain an amino acid (the "building blocks" of protein) called glutathione, which helps fight rheumatoid arthritis and Parkinson's disease, and also protects against heart disease and cancer. They are also rich in vitamin E, which is a powerful antioxidant (see page 19). Vitamin E is an important nutrient for good skin condition and protects against dryness and wrinkles, as well as helping wounds heal quickly with minimal scarring. Lastly, they are a good source of monounsaturated fat, which is also linked to protection against heart disease (see Olive Oil).

barley

Whole-grain barley—sometimes called "pot barley" —and other whole grains, such as rye and oats, contain a plant chemical called phytic acid, which has been shown to inhibit the growth of cancers by its antioxidant and immune-boosting properties. Whole grains are also high in total fiber and soluble fiber, which helps keep the digestive and circulatory systems healthy and to prevent heart disease and diverticulitis. Barley is particularly rich

See also:
▶ The diet plans, pages 28–31;
▶ Making sense of antioxidants, page 19;
▶ Phytochemicals, page 19.

in chemicals called protease inhibitors, which also have properties that combat cancers, including breast and bowel cancer.

black currants

Black currants are one of the richest natural sources of vitamin C, at around 130mg per 100g when stewed. Vitamin C is an important antioxidant that protects against disease, helps keep the immune system healthy, keeps the skin in good condition, and helps wounds and fractures heal. High levels of vitamin C are linked with the lowest risk of heart disease. It is best to get your vitamin C in its natural form rather than via supplements, which may not have the same protective effects. Black currants also contain other plant compounds, such as lutein (see Greens) and anthocyanins (see Blueberries), and the oil from their seeds has been shown to have anti-inflammatory effects, relieving arthritic and rheumatic pain.

blueberries

Discovered in recent tests to be the most powerful antioxidants of all—"mopping up" more free radicals than any other foods—blueberries have the strongest potential to prevent the negative effects of aging and the diseases of old age. It has been found that 100g a day can stimulate the growth of new brain cells and may help prevent memory loss. Blueberries are also rich in a plant chemical group called anthocyanins, which help oxygenate the skin and carry maximum nutrients to the surface to help keep it looking young. Many other red, purple, and blue berries have similar properties.

broccoli

Broccoli contains several important antiaging factors. It is high in antioxidant carotenoids, vitamin C and indoles, which help fight lung, breast, and colon cancers. It is rich in lipoic acid, a fatty acid linked with increased brain power and energy. It is high in the

compounds lutein and zeaxanthin, which help keep vision healthy (see Greens) and is also rich in fibre, and is a natural source of chromium, which helps regulate blood sugars. It is higher in vitamin E than many other vegetables, and vitamin E is linked with protection against Alzheimer's disease.

carrots

Carrots are richer than any other fruit or vegetable in carotenes – plant compounds which have a strong antioxidant effect that is important in helping to prevent cancers, particularly of the stomach and lungs. One study showed that carrot eating can cut the risk of lung cancer by half. Regular carrot intake can also help protect against macular degeneration and cataracts, can help minimize night blindness, and can reduce blood LDL cholesterol (the "bad" type). The carotenes in carrots also protect the skin from sun damage and skin cancers. Carrots should be eaten with a little oil or fat to help carotene absorption, and cooking them also helps.

celery

Valued across the world for years for its medicinal properties, celery is renowned for reducing blood pressure. This might be because of the plant chemical 3-n-butyl phthalid that it contains, as well as apigenin, one of the flavonoid plant chemicals. It is also an excellent source of potassium, a mineral that balances body fluids and can lower blood pressure in some. Celery also has anti-inflammatory properties and can help reduce pain from arthritis, as well as helping to beat fluid retention. One study found celery is among the vegetables most strongly linked with protection from bowel cancer.

eggs

Good-quality eggs (those that are fresh, organically farmed, and certified salmonella-free) are an excellent food, particularly as one gets older. They contain high levels of selenium—which might be lacking in the diet and has cancer- and heart-disease-fighting qualities—and iodine, which can help to promote healthy thyroid hormone activity. An underactive thyroid can cause tiredness and weight gain. Eggs also contain lecithin, a fatty substance that can help to prevent heart disease and gallstones. Eggs are rich in a variety of vitamins and minerals, including vitamin E and zinc—both in shortfall in many older people's diets—as well as the B group, which helps nerve health and stress, and protein. About four eggs a week are a good level to aim for (unless you have specifically been told to avoid cholesterol in your diet).

flax seeds

Flax seeds—sometimes called linseeds—are tiny golden seeds from the flax plant with several brilliant qualities. First, they are one of the few plant foods rich in the omega-3 fatty acid, alphalinolenic acid, which converts in the body to EPA and DHA, two fatty acids found only in oily fish. These fats have a host of important antiaging properties. They help to prevent blood clots, stroke, and heart disease; might help brain power and depression; can help arthritis and improve insulin sensitivity; and are vital in retaining smooth skin. Flax seeds also contain lignans—oestrogen-like plant compounds that might reduce menopausal symptoms in some women.

garlic

Fresh garlic contains several compounds, the most important of which is allicin. Allicin has been shown to have potent powers to protect against several health problems, including high blood pressure, viral and bacterial infections, candida, indigestion, stomach ulcers, and bowel disorders. Several studies have shown that it can reduce blood LDL cholesterol (the "bad" type) by about 12 percent, and inhibits new growth of plaque in the arteries that can lead to heart attack or stroke.

Garlic might also help to prevent cancers by inhibiting the growth of cancer cells and strength-·ening the immune system. Its high content of nitric oxide synthase might also help overcome male impotence. Onions, also from the same family, are rich in flavonoids and potassium, which can reduce blood pressure and keep the arteries healthy, and the onion family might also help to keep blood sugar levels even by regulating insulin production.

greens

Leafy dark green vegetables—such as Savoy cabbage, kale, and spring greens—are good sources of two carotenoids—lutein and xanthanin, which have been shown to help prevent age-related macular degeneration in the eyes, and cataracts, which are common in older people and can cause vision loss. Greens are also a good source of easily absorbed calcium to help maintain strong bones, while also being rich in potassium, which helps protect against calcium loss. Greens are also a good source of vitamins C and E, two strong antioxidants.

herbs

Several herbs are strong antioxidants even when used in the usual small amounts in cooking and salads. Thyme, oregano, rosemary, sage, basil, and cilantro all contain high levels of phytochemicals, which can help ward off heart disease and cancers. Oregano, for example, has forty times as many antioxidants as apples, according to the US Department of Agriculture, and in one study aged mice became more active when fed oil of thyme.

nuts

Nuts contain good amounts of magnesium, which is vital for energy levels. Magnesium can help maintain suppleness in the muscles, help avoid aches and pains, and might also help to prevent osteoporosis. Almonds, Brazils, and peanuts are good for helping to build or maintain muscle mass and they can protect against glaucoma, type-2 diabetes, and high blood pressure. Research has shown that just two 25g portions of fresh nuts a week reduced death from heart disease in male US doctors by up to 47 percent.

The fatty acids in nuts help to maintain soft, wrinkle-free skin, as well as sexual function, and nut flesh is a particularly good source of vitamin E (see Avocados). Brazil nuts are rich in selenium, an antioxidant mineral that might reduce the risk of some age-related cancers and breast cancer.

oily fish

Oily fish, such as salmon, herring, mackerel, and sardines, are the main source of the important fats called omega-3s (a branch of the polyunsaturated group of fats) in the diet. Such fish contain two particular omega-3 fats called EPA and DHA not found in any other foods. These special fats have been shown to have a wide variety of benefits to health, including protection against the decline of brain power and diseases of the brain, such as Alzheimer's and Parkinson's. They are also anti-inflammatory, helping to minimize the pain of arthritis and rheumatism. These oils can help all dry skin and allergic skin conditions. In addition they can help prevent blood clots, coronary disease, and stroke. (See also Flax Seeds.)

olive oil

Although olive oil, like other plant oils, is almost 100 percent fat, it is rich in nutrients and compounds that help protect against age-related disease. It is high in monounsaturated fats, which lower levels of the "bad" LDL cholesterol in the blood, while protecting the levels of "good" HDL cholesterol, and thus protect against heart disease and stroke. Olive oil also contains the compounds squalene and oleuropein, which are powerful antioxidants, protecting blood cholesterol from oxidation. This antioxidant effect might also reduce the risk of some cancers, particularly of the breast and colon. Top-quality, cold-pressed olive oils are the best to buy for health, as they contain greater amounts of the protective compounds.

onions

The onion family, including garlic and leeks, are good detoxifiers and are also antiseptic and antibacterial. Just 1g of onion a day is enough to help strengthen the bones, and the sulfur compounds contained in the onion family are also linked with protection against stroke, high blood pressure, heart disease, and cancers.

spices

Most spices are strong antioxidants and have a variety of beneficial effects. Ginger is an anti-inflammatory and can help ease the pain of both forms of arthritis. Chilies speed up the metabolic rate, thus helping both weight control and circulatory problems. Chilies also contain the plant chemical capsaicin, which is a great reliever of general aches and pains. Turmeric has been shown to reduce the brain plaques, which can cause Alzheimer's disease, and coriander seeds can lower high blood pressure.

soybeans

Soybeans contain high levels of plant estrogens and magnesium, both of which might help to minimize the symptoms of the menopause. Soybeans are high in soluble fiber, and have also been shown to help reduce the risk of heart disease. Soy protein helps build and maintain collagen and elastin, both important for maintaining skin in youthful condition. Lastly, soy contains good amounts of coenzyme Q10, the compound that has been demonstrated to have a beneficial effect on both energy levels and gum health.

tomatoes

Tomatoes are rich in the carotenoid lycopene, which offers protection against cancer and heart disease. Recent trials have found that women who eat a lot of lycopene have a reduced chance of getting both ovarian and breast cancer, while in men it helps prevent prostate cancer. Lycopene might also help to protect against osteoporosis. Tomatoes are again a good source of lipoic acid, which helps increase energy levels and improve brain power in some people. Small—cherry or similar—ripe tomatoes tend to contain the highest levels of lycopene and cooking them helps their absorption.

See also:
▶ Know your nutrients, page 18.

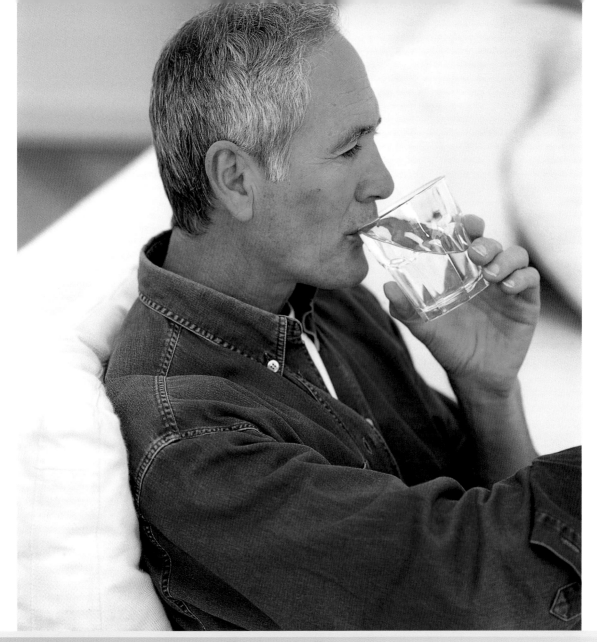

food for your **looks**

When the first signs of aging show in your looks, don't automatically think of cosmetics, lotions, potions, creams, gels, or drops as your main line of attack. If you want clear and smooth skin, shining hair, bright eyes, and teeth and gums to make you smile, the best way to achieve these is to eat the right diet. At any age, beauty really does start from within. There are foods that can help moisturize and plump your skin, and protect it from wrinkles, dryness, and sun damage; there are foods that will feed your hair and keep your eyes and mouth healthy—in fact, there is a food, or nutrient, for virtually every problem connected with your appearance.

skin

The early signs of skin aging include dryness and fine lines, both of which can be improved by simple dietary measures. Dryness is easily combated by a diet rich in unsaturated fats—particularly the longer-chain omega-6 essential fatty acids (for example, evening primrose oil) and long-chain omega-3 fats found mainly in oil fish. A daily supplement of both these oils should see improvement within two weeks. The US Department of Agriculture's updated dictory guide-lines for Americans recommend eating two 4-oz. portions of oily fish per week. NOTE: It is very important when eating a diet high in polyunsaturates also to eat plenty of antioxidant foods (see page 19) to make sure these highly unsaturated fats, which are unstable, don't oxidize in your body.

Also remember to drink plenty of fluids, as water literally helps to plump up the skin, avoiding that dried-prune look. In normal circumstances, eight glasses a day is about right.

It is also important to eat sufficient protein, which boosts the skin's collagen (to help plump up and pad out the outer layers of the skin) and elastin, which gives smoothness and elasticity. Lastly, to help avoid wrinkles and dryness, try to maintain a reasonable body weight and don't get too thin—a small layer of fat under the facial skin gives a smooth, healthy appearance, and often when people diet it is the face that loses the most weight.

A diet high in antioxidants (see page 19) is vital for good skin. It is thought damage to the collagen in skin by free radicals is one of the causes of tough and leathery skin. Antioxidants are also thought to help prevent the appearance of age spots or "liver spots" on hands and other body skin. These brown spots, like large freckles, which eventually can meld into one large brown area, are thought to be a by-product of the oxidation of polyunsaturated fats in the body, which produces a surplus of a substance called lipofuscin. Antioxidants, such as vitamins C and E, and especially anthocyanins (found, for example, in blueberries and other dark berries), can help prevent this buildup if eaten regularly. Antioxidants will also help prevent the oxidation of long-chain fatty acids after you've eaten them (see page 18).

Some minerals are vital for skin health—for example, zinc (found in good amounts in shellfish, whole grains, nuts and seeds) is vital for the manufacture of collagen and helps to speed up skin repair and renewal, and selenium (found in nuts, seeds, fish, and variety meat) is an antioxidant mineral that helps counter dry skin and free-radical damage.

If your skin is frequently exposed to outdoor weather, especially in the summer/around snow or water, or in the sun, you should eat plenty of foods rich in beta-carotene (one of the carotenoid group of antioxidants), such as carrots, mangoes, dark leafy greens, orange-fleshed melons and squashes, red peppers, broccoli, and tomatoes. Regular adequate beta-carotene intake offers the type of protection from sunburn afforded by a low-factor sunscreen (although, if out in the sun, you should still use a suncream, of course).

Although long-term use of beta-carotene supplements isn't recommended, as very large doses have been linked with possible increased risk of cancer, short courses (say, starting two weeks before a sunshine holiday) of 30mg/day for a maximum of four weeks will increase your skin's immunity to the aging and dangerous effects of UV rays. One study in 2002 showed also that supplementing with Vitamin C and E helps to guard against sunburn, although high doses of any vitamin supplement are not recommended. Lastly, there is some evidence that regular intake of foods containing the carotenoids lutein and zeaxanthin (see Eyes overleaf) might help to protect the skin in the sun.

thread veins—tiny, fine red veins that appear at

or near the skin's surface, particularly on the face, are a common problem in the 40s and after. Sun damage is a common cause of the appearance of these, so protect your face well from the sun, using a fake tan instead, if necessary. There is also a genetic predisposition to inherit them, and pregnancy can make them worse. They appear more obvious when the skin thins as we age, so see tips above for maintaining collagen. Some people say drinking alcohol and spicy foods makes thread veins worse, but I can't find any researched evidence for this.

eyes

Sparkling, bright eyes can take years off your looks. Although other factors—such as lack of sleep, being overworked or ill, or long hours at the computer—can make your eyes look tired and dull, a few changes in diet and lifestyle can improve them considerably.

Once again, a regular intake of the essential fatty acids (see Skin on the previous page) can help prevent some of the signs of eye aging, such as dryness (a frequent problem as we get older), which can lead to irritation, a "gritty" feeling, red eyes and more. Evening primrose oil, one of the long-chain omega-6 fats, may be particularly useful. You should also drink at least 8 glasses of fluid a day to make sure you are not dehydrated.

Dull eye whites can be encouraged to sparkle with a diet high in vitamin C, which will also help with redness. You also need to take regular outdoor exercise in the fresh air—it's surprising what a different this makes.

Red eyes and/or lids can be a sign of infection, so check this out with your doctor; otherwise it can be a sign of deficiency in vitamin B_2 (found in yeast extract, variety meat(s), seeds, legumes and nuts) or zinc (shellfish and whole grains).

hair

Poor nutrition and high levels of stress are two common causes of hair problems in midlife, particularly of hair loss and thinning hair. If you find this a problem, increase your intake of iron-rich foods, such as lean red meat and leafy dark green vegetables, as well as of zinc, calcium, selenium, and potassium.

You also need to take regular exercise to improve circulation. Hair loss in midlife women is often caused by a decline in estrogen levels, so it may be wise slightly to increase your intake of plant foods naturally high in estrogenic compounds, such as soy and other legumes, yams, and flax seeds.

Hair usually becomes drier as we get older, which can eventually lead to lack of shine and to brittleness—the hair doesn't look in good condition and can be hard to manage. Make sure you have adequate fats in your diet (especially the omega fats already discussed), along with the vitamin B group and vitamin C.

Graying hair is influenced by genetic predisposition rather than by diet, but the grayer the hair the more it may look dry or dull, so follow the tips above to make sure it stays shiny and in good condition. If stress is causing your hair to be in poor shape, see the tips on beating stress in Chapter 4 – Well-Being for Your New Life.

teeth and gums

Good teeth are important at any age, but especially now. A bad smile takes years off your face, and you want to feel confident that people are looking at a gleaming smile and good gums. Apart from regular cleaning and flossing, and possibly dental care and or surgery, there is much you can do via diet to help your smile look better.

Avoid a diet high in sugars and sugary foods (even including fresh and dried fruits), particularly those used as snack foods between meals. Sugars left in contact with your teeth and gums for hours at a time will help to produce cavities, tartar, and gum disease. Brush your teeth half an hour after any sugary food or drink. Note: We all need fresh fruit in our diets, so don't stop eating fruit, just remember to clean your teeth well afterwards.

Stained teeth aren't attractive, and stains seem to appear more readily as we age. Red wine and the tannins in tea are two major culprits in producing stains. If you like either or both of these (and both are healthy in reasonable quantities), use a stain-removing toothpaste.

Gum health is reliant not only on good hygiene, but also on good diet. You need plenty of vitamin C (fresh fruit and vegetables) to prevent problems such as redness or bleeding, and a very useful supplement is coenzyme Q10, which can achieve excellent results with problem gums after only a week or two of use.

hands and feet

For skin on the hands and feet, see Skin on the previous page. The hands are more prone to dryness than skin elsewhere on the body, probably because we put them in hot water and soap or detergent so much—so don't forget to wear protective gloves or use handcream afterward. Nails, in particular, will suffer if they are dry, splitting, breaking, and looking hard and unattractive.

The old wives' tale that gelatin is good for strengthening nails is NOT true. Nails consist mostly of protein, so a diet moderately high in protein is important to maintain their strength (lean meat, fish, dairy produce, nuts, legumes), concentrating on getting your weekly oily fish intake to help keep the nails supple.

If your nails are spoon-shaped (with a slight dip in the middle like the bowl of a fairly flat spoon), this indicates an iron deficiency, so increase intake of lean red meat, dark leafy greens, and whole grains. White spots on the nails indicate a zinc deficiency, so eat regular portions of shellfish, whole grains, lean red meat, and nuts and seeds. Nails take several months to grow from base to tip, so don't expect fast results.

diet plan for your 40s

The plan here is suitable for anyone—both men and women—in good health, and will help to improve your energy, looks, and ability to ward off the signs of aging. Before beginning, check the list of tips below:

tips

● I haven't given exact amounts as you should adjust portions to suit your own appetite and needs.

● Add as many leafy greens and/or salad vegetables (raw) to the plans as you like.

● Drink 8 glasses of water or equivalent a day—some of this can be in the form of weakish green, black, or milky tea. You can have 3 to 4 cups of weakish coffee a day, but stop drinking coffee by mid-afternoon and don't count this toward your day's fluid intake (although coffee isn't as dehydrating as is sometimes claimed). Avoid tea and coffee with meals, as they can hinder absorption of nutrients.

● It is best, nutritionally, to eat whole fruit rather than drink fruit juice, which is why there is not any juice mentioned on this plan. However, the occasional real-fruit smoothie or breakfast glass of juice is fine. Vegetable juice is an excellent drink and doesn't contribute to tooth decay/enamel erosion.

● When choices are given, or a food is unspecified ("portion of fresh fruit"), vary your choices as much as possible to improve your range of nutrient intake.

● Buy top-quality really fresh foods and take care with their cooking to preserve nutrients.

● If hungry between meals, snack on small handfuls of fresh seeds or nuts, or a small square of hard cheese.

day 1

breakfast
Fresh fruit salad
1 tablespoon sunflower seeds
1 teaspoon flax seeds
¾ cup low-fat yogurt with added bacteria

lunch
Smoked mackerel fillet open sandwich on rye bread
Side salad of red lettuce, onions, tomatoes, watercress, and olive oil Italian dressing
4 pieces of dried apricot

evening
Quick-fried sliced red peppers and bean-sprouts, with slices of lean beef tenderloin and broccoli florets, stirred in peanut or olive oil
Wholewheat egg thread noodles
Compote of poached fruits in season
Low-fat plain cottage cheese

day 2

breakfast
whole-grain breakfast cereal, with 2% milk
1 orange
5 whole Brazil nuts

lunch
Crab and avocado salad with shredded romaine lettuce
Whole-wheat bread with a little butter
Portion of fruit of choice

evening
Broiled chicken breast marinated in lemon juice and olive oil with thyme
New potatoes
Stir-fried shredded dark leafy greens
Carrots, steamed

day 3

breakfast

Boiled free-range eggs
Whole-wheat or rye bread with
a little low-fat spread
Pink grapefruit or fresh mango

lunch

Homemade or fresh chilled mixed vegetable soup (including, for example, onions, garlic, leeks, carrot, peas, and spring greens)
1 tablespoon grated Parmesan cheese
Wholemeal pita bread
Nectarine or plums

evening

Salmon fillet with good-quality pesto sauce basted
over top and broiled until cooked
Brown basmati rice
Salad of mixed fresh herbs and mixed leaves,
dressed in olive oil Italian dressing
¾ cup low-fat plain yogurt with live bacteria

day 4

breakfast

Whole-milk plain yogurt with live bacteria with
½ cup fresh blueberries and 1 handful luxury
muesli stirred in
Whole-grain bread and yeast extract

lunch

Good-quality canned tuna in spring water, drained
and mixed into a salad with arugula, tomatoes,
wedges of hearts of lettuce, sliced onions, and
drained canned cannellini beans
Apple or pear

evening

Whole-wheat pasta
Homemade tomato and basil sauce with soft goat
cheese stirred through
Large green side salad

day 5

breakfast

Traditional oatmeal with good-quality honey and
raisins stirred in; 2% milk
Apple

lunch

Organic baked beans in tomato sauce
Rye bread, toasted, with butter
Orange or papaya

evening

Casserole with Scotch barley, sweet potatoes,
onions, and cubed lean lamb
Steamed bok choy or spring cabbage
Low-fat plain yogurt with live bacteria with honey

day 6

breakfast

7oz. low-fat plain yogurt with live bacteria topped
with chopped fresh fruit, 4 teaspoons each
pumpkin seeds and flax seeds, and honey

lunch

Brie or Camembert cheese
Cherry tomato, arugula, and onion salad
Rye bread
Apple

evening

Roast chicken (lean only) torn into bite-size pieces
and stirred into a bulghar wheat salad with
chopped roast Mediterranean vegetables
(bell peppers, zucchini, red onion, eggplant)
Plain cottage cheese

day 7

breakfast

As Day 1

lunch

Omelet filled with mixed chopped fresh herbs
(thyme, mint, rosemary, oregano, chervil)
Rye bread with low-fat spread
Broiled tomatoes sprinkled with olive oil

evening

Cod or other white fish of choice, baked
Sliced yellow bell peppers and red onion, stir-fried
in olive oil and garnished with cilantro leaves
Baby new potatoes
Green beans

diet plan for your 50s

kick those bad eating habits
Eating more healthily can seem like hard work if you've been on a less-than-perfect diet for years. Use these tips to help make the change easier:

● Make changes gradually—particularly about including more legumes and vegetables in your diet. This will help you to avoid digestive problems, such as increased wind or heartburn.

● Eat regularly. The meal suggestions in the plans here will help keep your blood sugar levels even so you shouldn't feel hungry between meals.

● Don't be afraid to try new things.

● Cut down on sweet and salty flavors in your diet slowly. First cut out usage at the table, then reduce the amount you use in cooking and finally gradually give up high-salt, high-sugar foods such as potato chips, salted snacks, and candy.

● There is no harm in small amounts of treat foods and drinks, such as wine or good-quality chocolate. Don't feel guilty about these, but try to have them with or straight after a meal.

day 1
breakfast
Red and black berries topped with plain
    yogurt with added bacteria, sprinkled with
    sunflower seeds
Apple

lunch
Hard-boiled egg, sliced, with halved cherry
    tomatoes, sliced scallions, and fresh basil leaves
    served on dark rye bread, sprinkled with olive oil
Italian dressing

evening
Sweet potato slices layered with spinach and
    topped with a cheese sauce made using skim
    milk, sprinkled with extra cheese, and baked
    until tender and golden
Broccoli

day 2
breakfast
Bowlful of luxury muesli with 2 teaspoons
    flax seeds
Skim milk
Fruit of choice

lunch
Mackerel fillet in tomato sauce with a large
    mixed leaf and herb salad
Rye bread with low-fat spread
Red grapes or plums

evening
Griddled pork tenderloin
Steamed spring greens
Carrots
Snow peas
New potatoes

day 3
breakfast
Traditional oatmeal
    with honey and
    skim milk
Orange
5 almonds

lunch
Grated cheddar cheese, onion, and beet salad
    dressed in olive oil Italian dressing
Whole-wheat or rye bread with low-fat spread
Strawberries or raspberries

evening
Poached undyed smoked haddock with
    poached egg on top
Spinach
New potatoes

day 4

breakfast
Low-fat plain yogurt with live bacteria topped with
    any selection of red or purple fresh fruits
4 teaspoons *each* sunflower seeds and
    pumpkin seeds
5 walnuts

lunch
Organic baked beans in tomato sauce
Baked potato
Grated cheese
Green salad

evening
Lean roast beef or broiled steak
Savoy cabbage
Roast butternut squash
Fruit of choice

day 5

breakfast
Boiled egg
Whole-wheat bread with low-fat spread
Pink grapefruit segments
5 Brazil nuts

lunch
Slice of salmon and broccoli quiche made with
    whole-wheat flour
Large mixed salad containing a variety of
leaves and herbs
Plums

evening
Boneless chicken breast half stir-fried with
    chopped fresh chilies and ginger, bok choy, and
    bean-sprouts in peanut oil and a little soy sauce
Whole-wheat basmati rice
Fruit of choice with low-fat plain yogurt with live
    bacteria

day 6

breakfast
Special K with red berries
Plain fromage blanc
Whole-wheat bread with low-fat spread and
good-quality honey
Red grapes

lunch
Leek and garlic soup
Whole-wheat bread with butter
Parmesan cheese
Apple or orange

evening
Roast cod fillet
Green lentils cooked with onion and stock
Roast tomatoes with thyme

day 7

breakfast
As Day 1

lunch
Broiled goat cheese
Arugula salad
Cherry tomatoes
Blueberries

evening
Casserole of chickpeas, squash, tomato, broccoli,
    and boneless chicken thigh
Spring greens
Whole-wheat pasta shapes

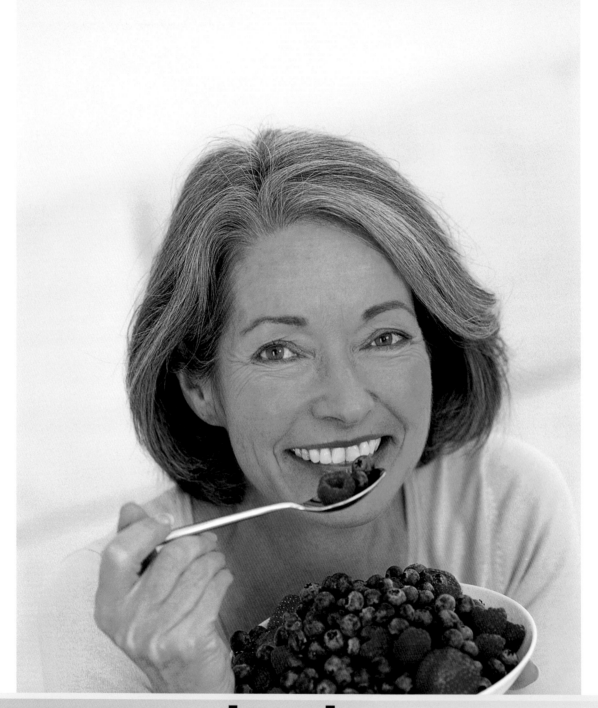

food for your **brain**

Brain power—including memory, concentration, and speed of communication—tends normally to be at its peak in youth and young adulthood, and can show signs of decline in the mid years. Much can be done to stop this downward spiral, however, and the right diet is a very important factor.

There is plenty of evidence to show that if you want to maintain all your "faculties" as you get older, there is no better time to begin making sure you eat well than right now. Several types of nutrients have been shown to help maintain your brain in "good working order" and prevent the brain diseases that most often attack in old age, including Alzheimer's and Parkinson's.

The first priority is to organize yourself a generally healthy diet, as outlined in the earlier parts of this chapter. For example, a diet low in fruit and vegetables and too high in saturated fat is strongly linked with a greatly increased risk of getting Alzheimer's disease later in life. There is also a link between the type of diet that is good for maintaining heart health and one that is good for the brain, and people with high blood cholesterol and/or high blood pressure (two markers for increased risk of heart disease) are also at higher risk of Alzheimer's. It appears to be the antioxidants in a healthy diet (see page 19) that have a particularly marked effect on reducing the risk of Alzheimer's. One large study reported in the Journal of the American Medical Association, in 2002, showed that volunteers with a high intake of vitamin C, vitamin E, beta-carotene, and dietary flavonoids were less likely to develop the disease.

Regular meals also predispose you to better brain power. There is much research to show that a good breakfast is important for brain function. A breakfast of whole-grain cereal and fruit has been found to improve memory by increasing your concentration, and the speed at which you process thoughts. This could be because breakfast gives you an all-important "shot" of glucose after a long night's fast, and the brain relies on glucose for its energy. It could also be that breakfast cereals are rich in vitamin B group, especially vitamin B_1, which has a special role in improving brain function.

brain food

The ancient belief that certain foods, notably fish, have extremely beneficial effects on the workings of the brain have recently received significant vindication from various scientific studies, and there seems to be a groundswell of public opinion in its favor. So much so that one UK supermarket chain announced in 2003 that sales of foods thought to be brain boosters were notably raised in areas with larger student populations, such as Oxford and Cambridge. Sales of fish, broccoli, asparagus, spinach, bananas, and all types of fresh fruit, and vitamin supplements soared during test times.

There is more on the power of fish for the brain in the later sections on Omega-3 fats and DMAE, and on broccoli and other vegetables (notably tomatoes) and fruits (notably blueberries), as well as turmeric and flax seeds, in the Top 20 Antiaging Foods on pages 20–3. We also look at brain-enhancing supplements overleaf.

Building on the foundation of a generally healthy diet and regular meals, all the following foods/nutrients have been shown to help improve brain functioning:

monounsaturated fats

During a 1999 Italian Study on Aging, it was found that a diet that was rich in olive oil (which is very high in monounsaturated fats) improved memory and helped prevent cognitive decline in old people, probably by maintaining the structure of the brain membranes. Monounsaturates are also to be found in good amounts in avocados and nuts.

omega-3 fats

There is much research to show omega-3-rich oily fish really does prove the old saying that "fish is good for the brain." Fish such as salmon, herring, mackerel, tuna, and sardines help to maintain the nerve function and the structure of brain cells, which contain a high concentration of these omega-3 fatty acids, and by helping the brain cells to communicate. The "active" omega-3 oils in fish are called eicosapentenoic acid (EPA) and docosahexenoic acid (DHA) and they are found in no other types of food at all. One 1999 review of studies on DHA found that a diet rich in this fatty acid does, indeed, improve learning ability.

The action of these oils is helped if the overall diet is low in saturated fat. Also a diet that is high in antioxidants (page 19) will make sure the omega-3 oils (which are part of the polyunsaturated group of fats) can work properly.

dimethylaminoethanol (DMAE)

All types of fish (not only oily) also contain a natural compound called dimethylaminoethanol (DMAE), which it is thought can improve your concentration and memory. Although there is little scientific evidence for its efficacy in this respect, a diet rich in fish might be worth a try.

vitamin E-rich foods

One 2002 study conducted by the US National Institute of Aging, published in the *Journal of the American Medical Association*, found that older people who had the highest intake of vitamin E were 67 percent less likely to develop Alzheimer's disease, while a Japanese study showed that brain disease in mice could be halted by injections of vitamin E. A third study by Harvard Medical School, published in October 2002 by *Neurology*, found that a diet rich in vitamin E can lower the risk of Parkinson's disease. In this study, more than 124,000 people were monitored for fourteen years. Vitamin E is to be found in olive oil and other plant oils, in avocados, nuts, seeds, egg yolks, and various vegetables and grains.

vitamins B$_{12}$ and folate

Low levels of these two B vitamins in the blood have been shown to increase the risk of Alzheimer's, according to a 2001 study published in the journal *Neurology*. Find vitamin B$_{12}$ in lean meat, variety meat, fish, eggs, and cheese, and folate in liver, legumes, fortified breakfast cereals, and leafy green vegetables.

red wine

One large Danish study carried out over thirty years recently found that drinking red wine can lower the risk of getting Alzheimer's disease by 50 percent. However, the amount of red wine needed is very small—one drink a week is enough, according to the research! (see box opposite).

coffee

Drinking moderate amounts of coffee throughout life might improve your brain power, two studies have found. One (published in the *European Journal of Neurology*) found that three to four cups of coffee a day consumed since the age of 25 led to a 60 percent reduction in Alzheimer's disease, when compared with people who drank one cup or less a day, while a study at the University of California found elderly women who had been lifetime coffee drinkers outperformed non-coffee drinkers in eleven out of twelve tests of cognitive power. Interestingly, in this latter research trial, the coffee helped only the women, not the men. It is thought this is because the ingredient in coffee held to be linked to improved brain power, caffeine, is processed in a different way in men and women.

supplements

Several supplements might improve brain power. Gingko biloba seems to increase capillary function and blood flow to the brain, which is an important factor in how the brain works (see also Exercise). Researchers at Tufts University, in Boston, found that people with the highest blood levels of folic acid had little or no memory loss after middle age.

Supplementation with zinc and iron is also recommended by additional US research that found men given a low-zinc diet for three weeks lost their ability to quickly recall specific words, and women with borderline anemia lost concentration and focus. Siberian ginseng might also affect the brain in a similarly positive way. The herb sage has also been used as a memory improver for many centuries, and sage tincture or pills can be tried.

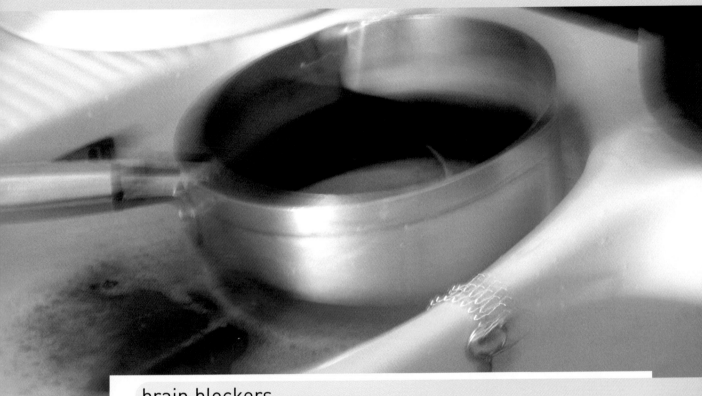

brain blockers

You can enhance the effect of the brain supernutrients listed opposite by cutting back on certain items in your diet, too.

sugar: Research conducted by the New York University School of Medicine has found that a diet high in sugar might encourage the hippocampus—the area of the brain that controls memory—to shrink. In tests, high blood sugar levels made participants perform badly in short-term memory tests. High blood sugar is also linked to insulin resistance (see page 16).

alcohol: Although small amounts of alcohol are good for health in older people in several ways, excess intake is not. Long-term high alcohol intake can affect short- and long-term memory—it appears to kill brain cells.

saturated fats: A high intake of these blocks the work of the polyunsaturated fats (omega-3s), which are important for brain health.

In addition, make sure your diet doesn't include added aluminum!

There is some research to indicate that ingesting aluminum might be linked with memory loss and/or Alzheimer's, so don't use aluminum pots and pans to cook food, especially acidic foods, such as fruit, as the aluminum easily leaches into the food.

food and **weight**

Very few people reach midlife without having put on some weight. For many of us, this produces feelings of failure and guilt as we try to battle with the extra pounds—all too often, unsuccessfully. So, here we examine all the middle-age weight dilemmas, sort out the truth from the fiction, and provide tips and blueprints for easier weight loss without too many sacrifices.

The American Obesity Association estimates that 127 million Americans are overweight, and 60 million of them obese or severly obese. In 2000, 33 percent of men aged 55 to 64, and 43 percent of women in the same age group, were obese.

If you are very overweight in your middle years, you are almost certain to be causing yourself health problems (if not now, then in the future) and may also be shortening your lifespan. According to one study published in the *American Journal of Epidemiology*, being overweight makes you about six "actual years" older than you really are, and, therefore, might shorten your life by a similar amount, while in the UK, Cancer Research UK puts the figure at seven years off an obese person's life, and the 2001 UK National Audit Office (NAO) report "Tackling Obesity in England" said that deaths linked to obesity shorten life by an average of NINE years.

the facts are these:
● Obesity is linked with a wide range of diseases and symptoms that are most common in people over 40. Heart disease, stroke, high blood pressure, some cancers, insulin resistance, type-2 diabetes, and osteoarthritis are the major ones, and it is now thought that overweight people are more prone to Alzheimer's disease. See the panel on page 39 for more detail on obesity/health links.

● Obesity is also responsible for a range of other problems, including social isolation, depression, and lack of self-esteem.

● Obesity is an increasing epidemic that has been put on a level with smoking as a cause of medical expenditure in the USA, and some estimates say that by the year 2020 most adults in the USA will be overweight or obese unless something is done.

Thus, if you want to lead a healthy life in midlife, and stay alive for your allotted span, you should tackle weight problems now rather than later. All the research shows that it IS possible to lose weight in middle age—and keep it off. And it is never too late to do so. Even as the pounds begin to come off, problems such as high blood pressure, type-2 diabetes, and angina can reduce in severity. And even if you are not severely overweight, keeping an eye on your calorie intake and lifestyle habits might prevent obesity in later years.

weight and good sense

Before you begin to try to shed pounds, you need to know if you really are overweight, for while obesity is linked with curtailed life, being too thin in your middle years is nearly as bad. That is because very low body weight is linked with greater risk of osteoporosis and low calorie intake can also be linked with a low intake of vital nutrients. Being too thin also predisposes you to dry skin and a greater chance of looking "wrinkly"!

First check your Body Mass Index. Find out your current weight (without clothes) and multiply it by 700. Now divide that figure by your height in inches, then divide again by your height in inches, and the result is your BMI.

If your BMI is 25 or under, you are not overweight. (If it is under 22 in midlife, you are bordering on thin.) If it is between 25 and 29 you are classed as "overweight," but for older midlife people, a BMI of 26–27 is not considered of great concern. A BMI of 30 or over is classed as "obese," and this is when the links with poor health and shorter lifespan really kick in.

You should also consider your shape. It is better to be a "pear" than an "apple," whichever sex you are. Fat stored around stomach/waist is linked with greater risk of heart disease, metabolic syndrome (opposite), and diabetes than fat on hips and thighs. A waist over 37 inches for men, or 31$\frac{1}{2}$ inches for women indicates a slightly increased risk, while over 40 inches for men and 34$\frac{1}{2}$ inches for women indicates substantially increased risk. After menopause, women are more prone to develop an apple shape, due to the reduction in female hormones, making the shape more "male."

the way to lose ...

If you do need to lose weight, you need to balance your food and drink (calorie) intake with the energy your body uses up. That normally involves eating and drinking a little less (of certain foods, see later) and doing a little more exercise on a regular basis. (For more information on exercise and weight reduction/control, see pages 80–85.) In midlife, even more than in your teens, 20s, or 30s, you need to achieve this balance by eating healthily and by avoiding fad or crash diets. Although it IS a longer affair to lose weight as you get older (see Myths, pages 40–41), the weight is definitely easier to control in the long term if you do things sensibly and make changes in your eating habits that you can stick with for the next twenty years or so.

wise dieting

● As much as possible, choose foods that are natural and healthy. It has been shown that diets that are regularly high in items such as baked goods, candy, desserts, potato chips, fast food, and highly processed foods of all kinds predispose you to weight gain and make it hard to lose weight.

● Don't reduce food intake too low. Eating just 100 calories a day less over a year would result in a loss of 10 pounds. Studies show weight lost slowly is less likely to come back.

● Choose foods low or moderate on the Glycemic Index. This measures how quickly foods are converted into glucose and absorbed into the blood. Foods high on the GI will be absorbed quickly and have you feeling hungry again before long, while low-GI foods keep blood sugar levels even and hunger at bay. A diet high in low-GI foods is especially important for diabetics and those with insulin resistance or metabolic syndrome (see opposite).

Low-GI foods All legumes, whole-grain pasta, whole-grain rye, Scotch barley, pearl barley; apples, dried apricots, peaches, cherries, grapefruit, plums, oranges, pears; avocados, zucchini, spinach, peppers, onions, mushrooms, leafy greens, leeks, green beans, lima beans, sprouts, snow peas, broccoli, cauliflower, tomatoes; yogurt, milk, nuts.

High-GI foods Glucose, sugar, honey, pineapple, raisins, watermelon, ripe bananas; baked/mashed potatoes, parsnips, cooked carrots, squash, rutabaga; brown/white rice other than basmati, rye crispbreads, whole-wheat/white bread, rice cakes, couscous; corn flakes, bran flakes, instant oatmeal, puffed cereal, wheat crackers, muffins, biscuits.

NOTE: The GI measures only carbohydrate foods, but both protein and fat foods reduce the rate of food absorption and so have a similar effect to low-GI foods.

● Choose a good balance of food types. A varied diet is important for health even while you are losing weight. Incorporate the healthy high-GI foods into meals that also contain low-GI foods, protein, and a little fat.

● Eat "little and often." Research shows that most people stick better to weight-loss plans if eating frequently, with no more than 3 hours between meals or snacks. This doesn't encourage overeating, if meals/snacks are small and healthy. "Little and often" has also been shown to reduce total calories eaten.

weight and health

Being overweight or obese in midlife is linked with several health problems. These are the main ones:

cardiovascular diseases
Excess weight, particularly around the midriff, is strongly linked with increased risk of heart and arterial disease and stroke, and of high blood pressure (hypertension), which can lead to cardiovascular disease. You need only be around 10 percent overweight to put yourself at higher risk of these problems. Abdominal fat is one of the five markers of insulin resistance syndrome (see below).

diabetes
Type-2 (non-insulin-dependent) diabetes, which used to be called "adult onset diabetes" because it becomes apparent most often in middle-aged people, has overweight as its main risk factor. Research shows that woman aged 35–55 have a forty times greater risk of type-2 diabetes if they are overweight, and it is believed that approximately 75 percent of cases of diabetes could be prevented by maintaining a reasonable weight with a BMI no more than 25. Overweight can also lead to insulin resistance, which is often a precursor of diabetes.

osteoarthritis
This is a very common complication of obesity and it is believed that the extra weight causes undue strain on the knee and hip joints and the back.

cancer
Obesity increases the risk of colon cancer by six times, while in women it increases the risk of breast cancer. One large study found that there was a 100 percent increased risk in women in their 50s, probably because the amount of the sex hormones estrogen and testosterone in the body are greater in obesity. Another study found that overweight increased the breast cancer risk by 40 percent in women aged 30–50, while overweight men increase their risk of prostate cancer by 20 percent. Cancer Research UK believes that one-eighth of all non-smoking-related cancers might be caused by weight problems, and the fatter you are, the greater the risks.

metabolic syndrome
Also called insulin resistance syndrome or syndrome X, metabolic syndrome is officially recognized as a medical condition, and someone is defined as having the condition if he or she meets at least three out of five criteria: central fat distribution (fat mainly concentrated around the abdominal area); high triglycerides (dangerous fats) in the bloodstream; low levels of the "good" HDL cholesterol in the bloodstream; high blood pressure; and high levels of glucose in the blood. Reducing weight and doing more exercise nearly always improve all these five symptoms.

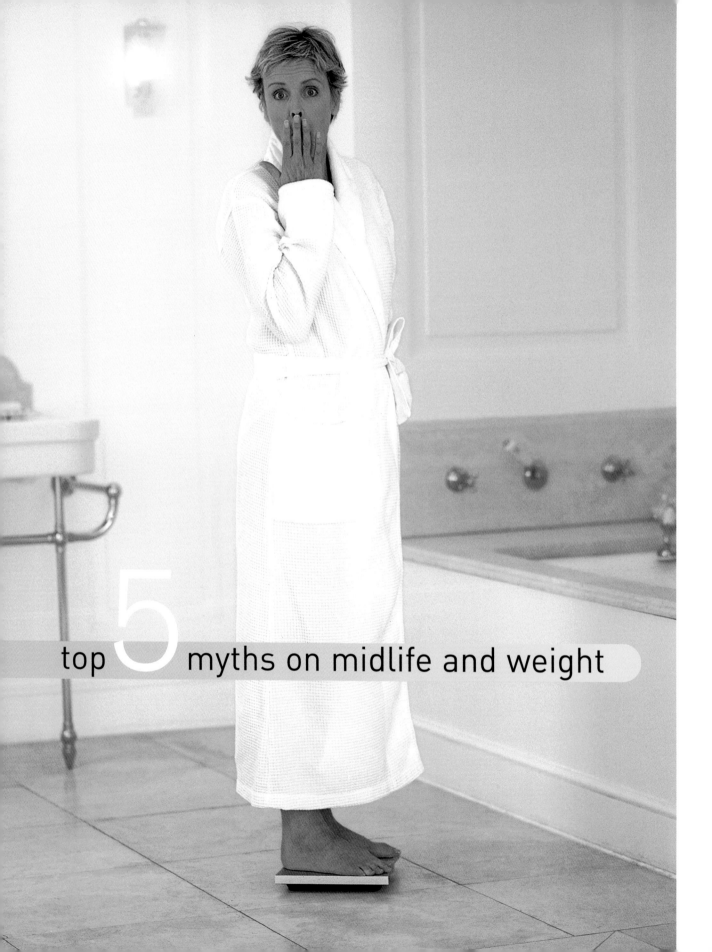

top 5 myths on midlife and weight

- **"It's my thyroid, doctor."** Although a small percentage of people do have problems connected with the thyroid gland (its main job is to regulate the body's metabolic system) that predispose them to put on weight, most of us don't. It is estimated that only 1–2 percent of people suffer from the medical condition hypothyroidism, symptoms of which can include weight gain, sensitivity to cold, tiredness, facial puffiness, and swelling of the thyroid in the neck. Diagnosis can be made by blood test, and treatment is usually with synthetic thyroid hormone.

  However, up to 10 percent of the population might have some symptoms of a sluggish thyroid without actual full-blown hypothyroidism, which might result in a borderline blood test. Females are more likely to have thyroid problems than men, and early middle age is a typical time when problems can become apparent. For the 90 percent of people whose thyroid is fine but they are overweight—look to lifestyle factors as the likely cause.

- **"I'm fat so my metabolism has slowed down."** People who are overweight often blame a slow metabolism for inability to lose weight, which is quite the reverse of the truth. All research shows that the fatter you are, the higher your metabolic rate. This is, quite simply, because the greater your body weight, the more work your body has to do to carry itself around and do everyday tasks. If you then lose weight, your metabolic rate will slow down as you diet. This is one reason people find it difficult to keep lost weight off. But research also shows that a previously fat, 140-pound person has a similar metabolic rate as an always-slim 140-pound person. In other words, dieting doesn't slow your metabolism per se—it is your new, lighter weight that is the culprit. If you want to stay slim, you will always have to eat less and exercise more than you did when you were fat.

- **"Middle-age spread is unavoidable."** Although research shows most people do gradually put on weight throughout the middle years, gaining on average 2 pounds a year, it is by no means inevitable. The main cause of this gain is that people tend to be less active as they get older, so that they burn up fewer calories in everyday life. Also, the proportion of lean tissue (muscle)—which naturally burns up more calories than other body tissue—diminishes. You can lose up to 5 pounds of muscle each decade after the age of 30, which, it is estimated, results in your needing about 100 calories a day less for every decade after that time. In other words, by the time you are 60 you will need 300 calories a day less than you did at 30.

  Both these causes of middle-age spread are largely preventable—keep active every day, and do weight-bearing exercise to maintain your lean tissue. These are discussed in detail in Chapter 2. Weight gain in the menopause is discussed on page 55.

- **"Yo-yo dieting over the years has ruined my ability to lose weight."** Yo-yo dieting (constantly losing weight then putting it back on again) can mess up the metabolism, up to a point, by repeatedly diminishing the body of lean tissue (muscle). When you diet, some of the weight you lose (about 15 percent) is muscle not fat. When you regain weight, unless you do a lot of exercise, the regained weight is more likely to be fat than muscle, then when you diet again, more muscle is lost, and if this pattern is repeated over the years, by midlife a yo-yo dieter may have much less metabolically active lean tissue than someone who has never dieted.

  However, if you begin exercising, particularly weight-bearing exercise, research shows you CAN replace lean tissue if you are determined, and you CAN become a reasonable weight and maintain that weight. Time and patience are the keys—your motto should be, "never yo-yo diet."

- **"It's healthy to be plump in middle age."** There is plump and plump. At 50, for example, it is probably wise to settle for a slightly higher weight than when you were, say, 25. This is because, firstly, being too thin can raise the risk of osteoporosis and can affect your hormones. To stay thin, most people eat a diet very low in fat, and this may make your skin and hair dry out—not a good side-effect if you value your looks. Fat has also been called "nature's HRT," helping to keep estrogen levels up during and after the menopause.

  However, a BMI over 26 or 27 is not healthy in middle age, so use your common sense. There is some evidence that fluctuating weight (for example, if you are a yo-yo dieter) is even less healthy than being overweight. So go for a sensible weight that you can maintain without too much difficulty.

Somewhere between 40 and 60, strange things sometimes happen to your body. You might not be particularly overweight, but parts of your previously fine anatomy gradually begin to let the rest of you down. The most common causes for complaint that I've come across are the appearance of cellulite and a stomach that refuses to stay in line with the rest of your profile. Both these problems seem to affect women more than men, although men aren't immune. Here we look at the causes, and at what can be done via diet to improve the situation.

cellulite and troublesome tummies

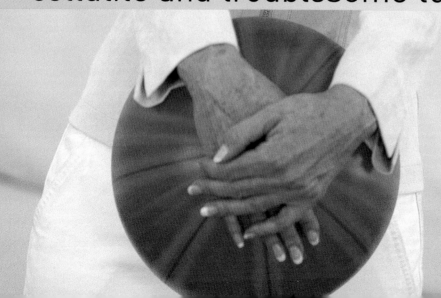

cellulite

The word "cellulite" is a lay description for layers of body fat that congregate just under the skin, most often around the hips and thighs of women, and which have a dimpled appearance. This fat is chemically the same as other body fat, but the cause of the dimpling seems to be that, in women, fat cells under the skin are grouped in sacs held in place with fibrous strands of connective tissue, which doesn't expand even when the sacs are bursting with fat—giving the "orange-peel" effect. In men, the connective tissue is differently formed; most men tend not to lay fat down on the hips and thighs, and what is there is covered with a firmer layer of skin.

Cellulite might make its first appearance on your body as you head toward midlife and might do less exercise, put on a few pounds, and the skin naturally begins to lose its firmness and elasticity.

What can be done? All research shows that most creams and potions on sale do little in themselves to cure cellulite. Indeed, the only treatments not related to diet or exercise that have been shown to have any effect are treatments with a powerful electric massager, called endermologie (available in salons only), and regular and vigorous massaging with a body brush, using any kind of lubricating cream.

There is also no proof whatsoever that a junk food diet, toxin-ridden diet, or any other particular diet, is the main cause of cellulite, unless such a diet causes you to put on weight, because even a few pounds overweight—if it tends to go to your lower body—can make cellulite dimples appear worse.

The best lines of attack are to stay slim and to take regular aerobic and strength-training exercise (concentrating on the lower body). For more on cellulite and exercise, see page 73. You might like to use the Detox Diet on pages 52–3, but again, in itself, the diet has no special magic powers to get rid of cellulite. The weight-loss plans that follow are a good starting point, although you shouldn't expect fast results. It can take several months.

tummy troubles

The main dietary cause of a stomach that seems to have a life of its own is bloating. This is usually due to fluid retention or gasses, and both problems can largely be corrected by diet (thank goodness!).

Fluid retention is usually caused by a diet high in carbohydrates, particularly refined white carbs, such as white bread, cakes, cookies and pasta, but also by sugar and sugary foods. These attract water as they pass through the system, and cause a lot of fluid to be retained (often around the stomach). As soon as you cut back on such items you will go to the bathroom more frequently and your stomach will shrink.

Another cause of fluid retention is a high-salt diet, so you need to cut back on salty foods like potatochips (double whammie these, as they are also a high-carb food) and savory snacks, and junk and processed foods of all kinds. Eating a diet rich in potassium helps eliminate fluid from the body – eat plenty of fresh fruit and veg. Other diuretic foods include many fresh herbs (particularly parsley) and salad vegetables, such as celery, and watermelons.

If bloating is due to gasses in the lower intestine, then try to find out what causes you to produce too much gas. Common triggers are legumes, cabbage, onions, dried fruits, dairy produce, wheat, yeast, coffee, and alcohol. Eliminate these one by one, as you don't want to give up healthy foods such as legumes or onions unless you have to. (TIP: If legumes or veg cause your bloating, cooking thoroughly and puréeing in a soup or casserole can often effect a cure.) Also eat "little and often" if prone to bloating caused by fluid retention OR gas. The Detox Diet on pages 52–3 should help with bloating as it incorporates all the dietary tips here. For more information on bloating, see Irritable Bowel Syndrome, page 192.

NOTE: A large stomach can also be caused by intra-abdominal fat, which can be caused by stress, menopause, or a genetic tendency to apple shape.

▶ **eat fat!** Very-low-fat diets are linked with depression, dry skin, and a range of health problems. Make sure to include some oily fish (for omega-3s), nuts and seeds (for omega-6s), avocado, and olive oil (for monounsaturates) in your diet on a regular basis. Small amounts of natural saturates such as butter, meat, and dairy produce, are also fine and help you to feel satisfied after a meal. Moderation is the key.

diets for weight loss

plan 1 For women and men with less than 14 pounds to lose

● This plan provides about 1,500 calories/day, which will result in steady weight loss for most women and for men with less than 14 pounds to lose, when combined with regular exercise (see Chapter 2).

● Every day you have an allowance of 1 cup skim milk for use in tea and coffee (up to 4 cups) or as a drink on its own. If you don't want this, have 1 tub (6-oz.) low-fat yogurt with live bacteria instead.

● You can also have unlimited green salad items and leafy green veg, such as lettuce, arugula, cucumber, scallions, red cabbage.

● Unlimited are any fat-free salad dressings, herbs, spices, vinegars, lemon juice, soy sauce, or Worcestershire sauce.

● You can have unlimited water, tea, and herbal tea.

● Every day you can have a medium glass of dry white or red wine or champagne. If you don't want this you can have a small chocolate wafer bar or any treat up to 100 calories.

monday
breakfast
2 whole-wheat biscuits with skim milk
    (extra to allowance)
1 peach or 2 plums
5 whole almonds and 5 walnut halves
snack
1 apple
lunch
1 medium breakfast bowlful of couscous
(reconstituted according to pack directions) tossed
        with ⅔ cup canned chickpeas, chopped red bell
        pepper, cucumber, and scallion, and 1 tablespoon
        olive oil Italian dressing.
6 oz. low-fat fruit yogurt, any flavor
snack
1 dark rye crispbread with 4 teaspoons vegetable pâté
evening
6 jumbo shrimp OR 5 oz. monkfish, cut into pieces,
marinated in Middle-Eastern harissa paste and broiled
1 cup cooked brown basmati rice
Large side salad with oil-free Italian dressing

tuesday
breakfast
1 tub (6-oz.) low-fat yogurt with live bacteria
    topped with 5 oz. mixed, chopped (as
    necessary) fresh fruit of choice, 1 tablespoon
    pumpkin seeds, and 4 teaspoons honey
snack
Apple
lunch
Take-away tuna-and-salad sandwich on
    whole-wheat bread
5 almonds
1 medium banana
snack
½ cup low-fat plain cottage cheese
evening
3½ oz. lean sirloin steak, sliced and stir-fried in
4 teaspoons peanut or olive oil with a 7-oz.
    selection of mixed vegetables, such as snow
    peas, corn kernels, carrot, or broccoli, sliced
    thinly as necessary, finished with a dash of chili
    sauce and soy sauce
7-oz. portion (cooked weight) whole-wheat egg
thread noodles

wednesday
breakfast
1 (1½-oz.) slice of whole-grain bread or
    toast with 2 teaspoons low-fat spread
    and honey
½ cup fresh orange juice
3½ oz. diet fruit yogurt
snack
1 pear or 2 plums
lunch
1 ready-to-eat pasta salad, any selection,
    containing not more than 350 calories
1 medium banana
snack
Handful (1 tbsp) sunflower seeds
evening
4-oz. salmon steak, brushed with a little
    good-quality pesto sauce and broiled until
    cooked through, 4 to 5 minutes
5 oz. new potatoes
3½ oz. green beans or broccoli
2 oz. baby corn cobs

thursday

breakfast

As Tuesday

snack

2 ready-to-eat dried figs

lunch

Greek salad made using 3 oz. crumbled feta cheese, crisp salad leaves, roughly chopped tomato or halved cherry tomatoes, cucumber, scallion or red onion, finely sliced red or yellow bell peppers, a few halved pitted black olives and 1 tablespoon olive oil Italian dressing

1 slice (1-oz.) whole-wheat or dark rye bread

snack

Apple

evening

3 oz. (dry weight) pasta of choice, cooked according to package directions and tossed with ½ cup good-quality tomato sauce for pasta

1 tablespoon shaved Parmesan cheese

Large green side salad with oil-free dressing

saturday

breakfast

½ cup no-added-sugar-or-salt luxury muesli

Skim milk to cover (extra to allowance)

1 nectarine or pear

snack

5 walnut halves

lunch

1 carton of any chilled ready-to-eat vegetable soup (without added cream), containing no more than 200 calories per carton

1 small whole-wheat roll with 1 teaspoon butter

snack

½ cup low-fat fromage blanc or cottage cheese

evening

7-oz. portion of cod fillet topped with 2 tablespoons good-quality Mediterranean sauce for pasta and baked at 350°F for 20 minutes or until the fleash flakes easily

5 oz. new potatoes

½ cup shelled peas

½ cup broccoli florets

1 small banana

friday

breakfast

½ cup low-fat fruit fromage blanc or cottage cheese topped with ⅔ cup sliced strawberries or other berries of choice, such as blueberries or raspberries

1 slice (1-oz.) whole-grain or dark rye bread with 1 teaspoon low-fat spread and honey

snack

5 whole almonds

lunch

2 oz. dressed crab tossed with 1 tablespoon low-fat mayonnaise mixed with 1 tablespoon low-fat plain yogurt and a little lime juice and rolled in 1 tortilla with chopped salad items of choice

1 slice cantaloupe melon or 1 peach

snack

1 dark rye crispbread with 4 teaspoons vegetable pâté

evening

6 oz. skinless chicken breast half, cut into bite-size pieces, marinated in lemon juice with crushed garlic, chili, and fresh cilantro leaves plus seasoning to taste, then threaded on a kabob skewer and broiled for 8 minutes, turning once, until cooked through

1 cup cooked brown basmati rice

Tomato and onion side salad with 1 tablespoon olive oil Italian dressing

sunday

breakfast

2 (1-oz.) slices of extra-lean Canadian bacon, broiled and served with 1 medium poached egg, 1 broiled tomato, and 2 tablespoons low-sugar, low-salt baked beans in tomato sauce

1 slice (1-oz.) whole-wheat bread with 1 teaspoon low-fat spread

lunch

5 oz. roast chicken breast (no skin)

5 oz. new potatoes

Steamed greens

Steamed carrots

Fat-skimmed gravy

1 cup mixed berries topped with 1 tablespoon plain yogurt and 1 teaspoon sugar

evening

Sandwich 2 slices (1-oz. each) whole-wheat bread with 2 teaspoons low-fat spread, 3½ oz. tuna in spring water, well drained, salad items of choice, and 4 teaspoons low-fat mayonnaise.

1 apple or orange

diet plan 2

For men with more than 14 pounds to lose and women with more than 42 pounds to lose
This plan is based on getting about 1,700 calories a day. The daily allowances and so on. are the same as for Plan 1. If you find you are not losing weight at a rate of at least a pound per week on this diet, change to Plan 1.

monday
breakfast
¾ cup low-fat yogurt, any flavor, with 4 teaspoons sunflower seeds sprinkled over
1 medium banana
1 satsuma or kiwi fruit
snack
5 whole Brazil nuts
lunch
Avocado salad: mix 1 small sliced ripe avocado with mixed salad leaves, sliced red onion, halved cherry tomatoes, and 4 teaspoons pine nuts, with 1 tablespoon olive oil Italian dressing
1 small whole-wheat roll
snack
1 dark rye crispbread with 4 teaspoons vegetable pâté
evening
5 oz. lamb steak, broiled
1½ cups couscous
3½ oz. broccoli

tuesday
breakfast
1 slice (1½ oz.) whole-wheat bread, toasted and topped with ⅔ cup low-sugar, low-salt baked beans in tomato sauce
½ cup fresh orange juice
snack
5 almonds
lunch
1 baked potato (8 oz.) topped with 3½ oz. drained tuna in spring water mixed with 1 tablespoon low-fat mayonnaise and a little lemon juice and pepper
Large mixed side salad with 1 tablespoon olive oil Italian dressing
1 apple or pear
snack
½ cup diet fromage blanc or cottage cheese
evening
Omelet made from 2 extra-large eggs, cooked in a nonstick pan with 2 teaspoons peanut oil, filled with a mixture of thinly sliced button mushrooms, fresh bean sprouts, cilantro leaves, and a dash of light soy sauce
¾ cup cooked and chopped new potatoes, sautéed in 2 teaspoons peanut oil
⅔ cup petit pois
3½ oz. steamed bok choy

wednesday
breakfast
Milkshake: blend ¾ cup 2% milk with I small peeled banana, roughly chopped, ⅔ cup sliced hulled strawberries, and 2 teaspoons honey; serve chilled
1 slice (1 oz.) whole-wheat bread with 1 teaspoon low-fat spread and reduced-sugar jam
snack
5 Brazil nuts
lunch
1 wholemeal pita bread or wrap filled with 1 heaped tablespoon good-quality hummus, served with a selection of raw vegetables, such as carrot, celery, bell peppers, and tomato
1 apple
snack
½ cup low-fat fromage blanc or cottage cheese
evening
Chicken Caesar salad: Cook 1 boneless chicken breast half and remove skin, slice and place on a large bowlful of torn romaine lettuce leaves dressed with a good-quality Caesar salad dressing; top with baked croutons
1 orange

thursday

breakfast

½ cup luxury muesli with 1 tablespoon sunflower seeds and 1 chopped apple prinkled over

Skim milk to cover (extra to allowance)

snack

1 dark rye crispbread with 2 teaspoons Marmite

lunch

1 cooked smoked mackerel fillet (3½ oz.)

1 slice (1 oz.) whole-wheat bread with 2 teaspoons low-fat spread

Large green side salad with oil-free dressing

1 medium banana

snack

Apple

evening

3½ oz. ball mozzarella, thinly sliced and interleaved with l thinly sliced tomato in an individual gratin dish, with fresh basil leaves sprinkled over and 1 tablespoon olive oil Italian dressing plus a dash of balsamic vinegar; place under a hot broiler for 2 minutes, or until the cheese is partially melted. Serve with 1 slice (1½ oz.) crusty whole-wheat bread to mop up the juices

1 satsuma or kiwi fruit

friday

breakfast

2 whole-wheat biscuits, such as Weetabix, with skim milk (extra to allowance)

1 peach or nectarine

1 slice (1 oz.) whole-wheat bread with 1 teaspoon low-fat spread and honey

snack

Small handful pumpkin seeds

lunch

2 slices (1 oz.) dark rye bread with 2 teaspoons low-fat spread, filled with 1 large hard-boiled egg, sliced, 2 oz. shelled shrimp, 4 teaspoons low-fat mayonnaise, and salad of choice

1 apple

snack

¾ cup pot low-fat yogurt with live bacteria

evening

Vegetable curry: Cook ⅔ cup potato chunks and ⅔ cup butternut squash chunks until almost tender, then stir in a nonstick pan with 2 teaspoons each peanut oil and curry paste, then add ¼ cup vegetable stock, 2 oz. spinach leaves, and 2 tablespoons cooked chopped green beans. Cover and simmer 20 minutes, then stir in 2 tablespoons low-fat yogurt with live bacteria. Serve on ½ cup cooked basmati rice

saturday

breakfast

As Monday

snack

5 walnut halves

lunch

chilled ready-to-eat vegetable soup (without added cream), containing no more than 200 calories

1 small whole-wheat roll with 1 teaspoon butter

snack

4 dried ready-to-eat apricot pieces

evening

1 medium trout, broiled until cooked through

2 tablespoons toasted almonds

5 oz. new potatoes

3½ oz. green beans

½ cup sweetcorn kernels or peas

Lemon wedge, to garnish

sunday

breakfast

2 large eggs, poached

1 slice (1½ oz.) whole-wheat bread, toasted with

2 teaspoons low-fat spread

½ cup fresh orange juice

snack

5 walnut halves

lunch

3 traditional Scottish oatcakes

2 tablespoons good-quality guacamole

Tomato and red onion side salad with oil-free dressing

evening

5 oz. lean roast beef OR trimmed steak, broiled

1 baked potato (7 oz.)

Large portion steamed greens

Steamed carrots

Fat-skimmed gravy

⅔ cup portion of fresh fruit salad with

1 tablespoon plain yogurt

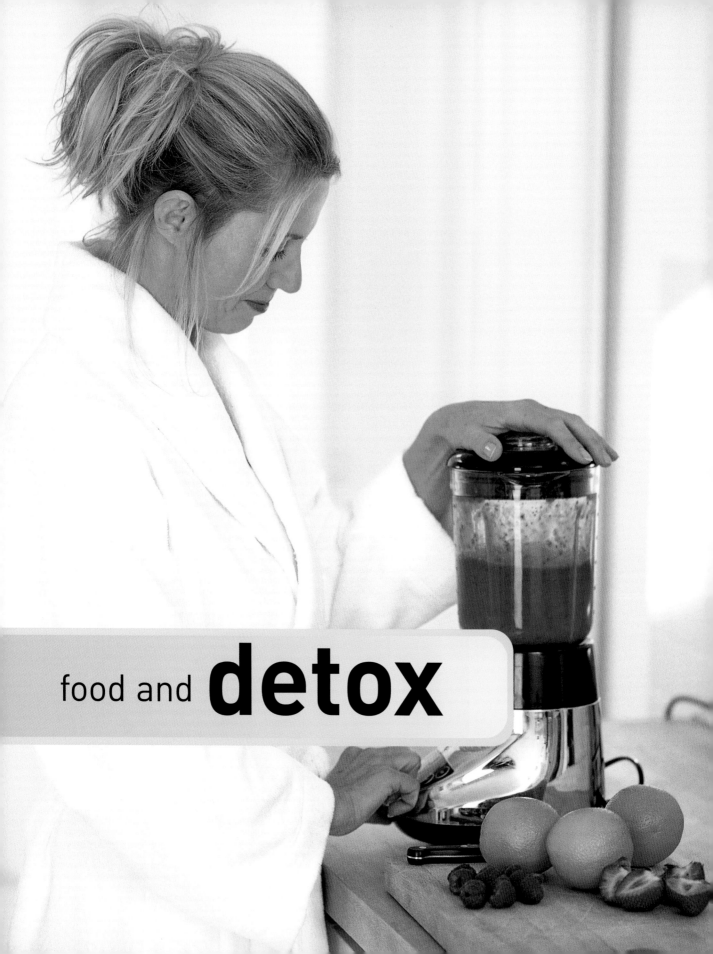

food and **detox**

If you're not exactly ill, but nevertheless feeling a bit under par—perhaps tired all the time, lethargic, lacking in your old sparkle, or zest for life—you might have considered doing a "detox" program. After all, everyone else seems to have done it. Here we ask, is a detox really for you? And provide all the answers...

There's probably been more nonsense talked and written about the mysterious process of "detoxing" than almost any other diet or health matter. Here are the answers to all your questions.

what is a detox?

A detox is the process of ridding your body (and, some say, your mind, perhaps even your whole life) of negative and/or unnecessary baggage and/or pollutants that are creating unwanted effects. A dietary detox (what mainly concerns us here) generally takes the form of switching to a diet high in the foods and drinks that will actively promote a detox effect, while avoiding the foods and drinks that are negative in this respect. What exactly these diet items consist of is the subject of much debate among "detox" experts.

does a detox diet work?

It is certainly possible to feel better in several ways at the end of a detox—for example, most people report feeling less tired and much less lethargic, with increased energy. Many report better skin and brighter eyes, and almost all tend to lose weight.

how does a detox work?

There are many claims made for how and why detoxes work to make you feel better and look better, but most claims are based on the idea that chemicals in the chosen detox foods help purge your body of "toxins," such as heavy metals, drug residues, and other pollutants, and that the banned foods are those which, in one of several ways, might encourage toxicity in your body.

In truth, a good detox diet is simply a high-vitamin, high-antioxidant short-term diet that increases your fluid, fruit, and vegetable intake and reduces the amount of highly processed foods you eat. All detoxes require you to give up a long list of foods, the usual no-nos being those containing additives, residues, salt, added sugar, wheat, and animal fat. The less healthy your predetox diet is, the more likely you are to feel better after the detox, but few of the individual foods on a detox have any particularly miraculous properties; it is a combination of factors that produces results. Indeed, many of the foods that are often banned—such as bread, potatoes, meat, and fish—are, or can be, perfectly healthy foods for most people. Their exclusion may be more a matter of opinion than science.

are there any negative side effects of detoxing?

In the short term, many people report headaches, probably due to withdrawal symptoms from caffeine, or even from a food to which you may be mildly intolerant (such as dairy produce or wheat). Others report a breakout of acne or blotchy skin, which could be due to a high intake of fruits, or, as many detox experts claim, is an indication of the "poisons" eliminating themselves from your body. Some people actually feel more tired in the first days of a detox. All these symptoms tend to disappear about 3 to 5 days into the detox.

when the detox is over, what should I do?

Gradually begin including a little more food in your diet, adding portions of healthy foods that your detox has avoided, such as root vegetables, fish, and poultry. If particular problems have cleared up on your detox—irritable bowel syndrome, for example—then reintroduce foods one by one to see if you can find the culprit. For most people, however, a balanced diet, including a wide range of foods, is healthiest in the long term, so don't avoid reintroducing ordinary foods unless there's good reason. Try to steer clear of highly processed and "junk" foods now your body has become used to living without them, and go easy on alcohol and caffeine.

1 are you:
a) **Overweight?**
b) **About the right weight?**
c) **Underweight?**

2 do you eat highly processed foods, white carbs, "junk" foods:
a) **Every day?**
b) **Fairly frequently?**
c) **Rarely or never?**

do you need a detox?

If you're still wavering about whether you should try a detox or not, answer these ten questions and then check your score ....

how long should a detox last?

Some people do a 2- or 3-day detox once a month, others do a week every 3 months, others a month once or twice a year. My own experience shows that a "grade-1" detox should only be carried out for up to a week, while a more moderate detox can be beneficial for a month or so.

Doing a detox for just a day or two is really a short-term crash diet by any other name, and while it may help you to feel less guilty about pigging out last weekend, is unlikely to achieve a great deal in the way of ridding your body of pollutants. Pollutants, such as heavy metals and drug residues, are stored in body fat, which cannot be got rid of in a few days, as we are all painfully aware!

3 do you drink alcohol:
a) **Every day?**
b) **Several times a week?**
c) **Rarely or never?**

4 thinking about your lifestyle, your job, your overall stress levels, are you:
a) **Living a very stressful life?**
b) **Stressed sometimes, but not all the time?**
c) **Rarely stressed?**

5 on most days, do you feel:
a) **Tired all the time and very lethargic?**
b) **Usually OK, but get tired easily?**
c) **Full of energy and enthusiasm?**

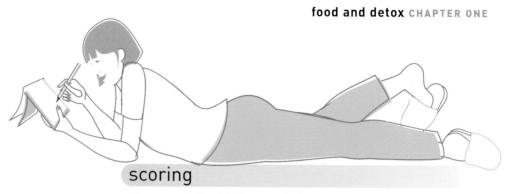

6 how strongly do you feel you need to change and/or refresh your life?
a) Very strongly?
b) Moderately so?
c) Not at all?

7 compared with other areas of your life, how much attention have you paid recently to your diet:
a) Hardly any?
b) A fair amount of attention?
c) A great deal?

8 How would you rate the condition of your skin (appearance, texture):
a) Very poor?
b) Average?
c) Very good?

9 do you have gum problems, such as bleeding or inflammation:
a) All the time?
b) Now and then?
c) Rarely or never?

10 looking at your eyes in a mirror in daylight are they:
a) Tired, bloodshot, or tinged yellow?
b) Not too bad for your age?
c) White whites, sparkling, and alert?

scoring

Give yourself 3 points for every A, 2 points for every B, and 1 point for every C. Add up your total.

If you scored 25 to 30:
You are in dire need of a mind and body detox. You need to recognize you and your body are as important as, if not more important than, any other factors in your life. You might feel you haven't time to put yourself on a detox program, but you need it more than most. Make the time—start the detox program overleaf, either for a long weekend or take a week's vacation and do it then. While doing it, try to be self-aware and learn ways to treat yourself as you deserve to be treated. Couple your diet detox with a gentle exercise program (see Chapter 2) and plenty of relaxation. Try to build the things the detox teaches you into your everyday life on a permanent basis.

If you scored 11 to 24:
You probably eat reasonably well and feel you have your life under control—but take care; in midlife it is harder to maintain optimum levels of energy and health unless you spend real time understanding the changing needs of your body. You can benefit from a gentle detox—try the program overleaf (moderate version) for a week and note the differences in how you feel. A week like this once a month will probably produce more benefits and help you change your food choices for the better every day of the year.

If you scored 10 or under:
You probably are an extremely healthy and perfect example of how to manage yourself and your life as you head into middle age—in which case, very well done. Few people live an exemplary life, even if they know what they should be doing! It is unlikely you need a detox diet—in fact, if you are underweight, a serious detox is not for you, as the calorie content is almost always low.

A word of warning: if anyone has ever described you as a "health fanatic," or perhaps a "health-food freak," or if you agree with either description of yourself, take care—there is evidence it can be as unhealthy to be obsessive or borderline obsessive about your health regime as it is to be a couch-potato junk-food junkie!

the detox diet

The 7-day Grade-1 detox plan here can also be used for just three or four days if you prefer. (Pick the first three or last four days.) The moderate detox (bottom of the opposite page) can be done for one week up to six times a year, two weeks up to four times a year, or for a month up to twice a year. Alternatively, devise your own plan using the list of "dos' and don'ts" opposite.

instructions

● Follow the Grade-1 diet for up to one week only and for no more than six times a year.

● Drink 8 glasses of water daily (or replace some of the water with green or tea with milk), spaced out evenly throughout the day. On rising every day, have a drink of hot water with the juice of half a lemon and 2 teaspoons honey.

● Have two between-meal snacks daily, one of 5 to 10 fresh almonds, Brazil nuts, or walnuts, the other of I tablespoon pumpkin or sunflower seeds.

● All salad leaves are unlimited.

● Try to eat all organic food.

● Have portions according to your appetite, size, and exercise levels.

● Avoid long periods of vigorous exercise while on the Grade-1 detox. (It doesn't provide enough calories.) Stick to moderate periods of aerobic exercise like walking, breaststroke swimming, or moderate-paced cycling, and other forms of exercise, such as yoga or stretching.

● Support the detox with regular baths or showers, body-brushing, and at least an hour a day of "self" —meditation, massage, and so on.

day 1

breakfast
Fresh fruit salad (no added sugar; use fresh fruit juice or water to moisten)

lunch
Salad of mixed dark-green and red leaves with a handful of fresh herbs of choice (chopped or torn), with olive oil Italian dressing, and $\frac{1}{2}$ avocado sliced in
Slice of watermelon

evening
1 medium bowl homemade lentil soup (using brown, green, or Puy lentils, salt-free veg stock, and chopped onion—simmer for 45 minutes, then purée if you prefer and reheat)
1 apple

day 2

breakfast
Fruit smoothie made by blending a selection of soft fruits (such as berries, bananas, mango, peach, or nectarine) with some water to make a thick drink; add honey if you like

lunch
2 tablespoons homemade or best-quality hummus
2 salt-free brown rice cakes
Large salad of leaves as Day One (exclude the avocado), sprinkled with 4 teaspoons pine nuts

evening
1 medium bowl homemade vegetable soup, using any orange or red veg (chop, simmer in salt-free vegetable stock for 45 minutes, then purée, if you prefer, and reheat)

day 3

breakfast
2 tablespoons wheat-free, oat-based muesli with 1 chopped apple and soy milk
1 slice of watermelon

lunch
1 bowl of vegetable soup as Day 2
2 unsalted brown rice cakes

evening
Large sliced tomato, red onion, and basil salad with 1 tablespoon olive oil Italian dressing beaten with 1 tablespoon good-quality guacamole and sprinkled with 4 teaspoons linseeds

day 4

As Day 1

day 5

breakfast

1 apple and 1 orange, each segmented and arranged with 1 small sliced banana; drizzle with 2 teaspoons honey

lunch

1 bowl of lentil soup as Day 1
1 medium slice dark rye bread

evening

Salad of cucumber, peppers, tomato, red onion, fresh cilantro leaves, and black olives dressed with 1 tablespoon olive oil mixed with 4 teaspoons balsamic vinegar and black pepper
5 Brazil nuts

day 6

breakfast

As Day 2

lunch

Purée of cooked lima beans with lemon juice, olive oil, and black pepper, with 2 unsalted brown rice cakes
Large mixed salad of choice with olive oil Italian dressing
1 apple

evening

Selection of Mediterranean veg (such as zucchini, eggplants, red onions, tomatoes), sliced, drizzled with olive oil and black pepper, and roasted for 45 minutes with a few whole garlic cloves. Drizzle more oil and lemon juice over, mixed with tahini to serve
1 slice of dark rye bread

day 7

As Day 3

Grade-1 detox

Follow this list of foods to use and foods to avoid to devise your own detox. The section at the bottom shows add-ons for longer-term use (see the introduction).

foods to go for

All fruits (including a few dried fruits, if you like, but make sure they are organic), preferably raw, but occasionally lightly cooked is fine. Fresh fruit smoothies are preferable to extracted juices as they retain more nutrients, but juice is fine now and then.

- All vegetables, raw or lightly cooked (for example, steamed or stir-fried in olive oil), or used in a soup or casserole. All salad items should be raw

- All legumes (such as lentils, chickpeas, navy beans, and black-eyed peas), dried and cooked, or use good-quality canned in water; sprouted legumes, soymilk

- All fresh herbs, such as parsley, rosemary, thyme, sage, chervil, basil, cilantro, and dill. All fresh spices, such as ginger, and dried whole spices, such as black pepper

- Good-quality olive oil, peanut oil, walnut oil, and sesame oil

- Fresh nuts and seeds, organic peanut butter, and tahini

- Brown basmati rice, brown unsalted rice cakes, dark rye bread, and rolled oats

- Top-quality single-source organic honey, preferably manuka

- Salt-free, artificial-additive-free vegetable stock

foods to avoid

- Meat, poultry, fish, dairy produce, eggs

- Sugar and processed carbohydrate foods, including white bread, and white rice

- Highly processed foods containing additives; long-life, heat-treated foods

- Wheat and wheat-based products, including wheat bread, wheat breakfast cereals, cakes, cookies, pastry, and wheat pasta

- Foods with added salt. If doing a lot of exercise in hot weather you might need a mineral-balanced energy drink to supply essential body salts

- Alcohol and caffeine-rich drinks, such as coffee, strong tea, cola; all carbonated drinks and diet drinks

Moderate detox Add these foods into your menus on the Grade-1 detox for a more gentle regime, higher in calories and protein (all foods should be organic): ● Chicken and game ● White fish, oily fish ● Low-fat yogurt with live bacteria ● Up to 2 slices of dark rye bread a day in addition to those listed in the 7-day diet.

food for
menopause

There is much women can do through diet to combat the side effects and possible negative health effects of menopause. As worries over taking Hormone Replacement Therapy (HRT) seem to escalate, with two out of three women giving up HRT drugs within a year, dietary intervention might be the sensible way to go. On these pages we look at the many links between diet and menopausal health, as well as examining the truth behind the headlines, and finally there is a blueprint menopausal diet.

The time around and after the female menopause is linked with several health problems, some potentially serious. The feature on Menopause and Andropause in Chapter 4—Well-Being for Your New Life—discusses the menopause in more general terms. Here we look at whether or not your diet can minimize the risks and influence the outcome.

weight gain
As we saw earlier in this chapter, too much weight gain in midlife is associated with an increased risk of health problems. Very many women report that they gain most weight during and immediately after menopause. Until recently, most studies on the subject came to the conclusion menopause itself wasn't responsible for this increase, and weight gain was simply because women at this time exercised less, or that it was a continuation of the gradual decline in metabolic rate that happens to us all after about 35.

Two more recent studies indicate women ARE right when they say that menopause piles on extra pounds even if they eat no more and exercise just as much.

One found that menopausal women put on about 2 pounds extra a year without any changes in diet or lifestyle, due to a sudden decrease in metabolic rate, while a study published in the *Journal of Clinical Endocrinology* found that changes in the way body fat is metabolized predisposes post-menopausal women to gain fat around their stomach and bottom.

In view of these findings it seems even more important to eat a healthy diet, moderate in calories and fat, to try to limit the amount of weight that is gained. Advice on menopause and exercise is on page 177.

bone loss
The demineralization of your bones speeds up at menopause by 600%, due largely to the huge decrease in the hormone oestrogen circulating in the body, and this may result in osteoporosis later in life. Indeed, one in five people over the age of 60 have the disease.

Much can be done to protect the bones via diet (see Around 50, page 16). There has been a great deal written in the past few years about using plant oestrogens to maintain bone density in the menopause. These phyto-oestrogens have a mildly oestrogenic effect within the body which, some experts think, will replace natural oestrogen at the menopause and after.

However, although short-term studies of high plant oestrogen diets suggest a small protective effect in the spine, there is little scientific evidence in humans for their usefulness. Trials using rodents, on the other hand, have consistently shown that diets high in soya or other isoflavones (a group of phyto-oestrogens) DO help prevent bone loss.

The COT concludes that more human trials need to be

done, while the UK Food Standards Agency (FSA) advises that the amount of plant estrogens needed in the diet to have even a small effect on the bones would be so great that it isn't an effective treatment for osteoporosis. That said, a 2002 scientific study reported in the *Journal of Bone and Mineral Research* found that supplementation with 54mg a day of genistein (a type of isoflavone) was as successful as HRT in maintaining bone health.

It might soon be proved supplements are the answer. In the meantime, a diet rich in phytoestrogens MIGHT help your bones and could be worth trying, especially if osteoporosis runs in your family. However, if you have—or are at risk from—breast or other hormonal cancers, the FSA advises you DO NOT eat a high-estrogenic diet or take supplements.

cardiovascular disease (CVD)

Once women have been through menopause, their risk of contracting any of the diseases of the cardiovascular system increases to the same level as that of men. This is because they no longer have the protection the female hormones appear to offer. A diet rich in antioxidants (see page 19), omega-3 fats, fruit, vegetables, whole grains, and legumes, and maintaining a reasonable weight, can offer protection against CV diseases. Regular intake of soybeans or soy products offer protection from heart disease. In the United States, manufacturers are allowed to make such health claims on labeling. Supplementation with isoflavones extracted from soybeans doesn't show similar levels of protection.

cancers: After menopause, there is increased risk of breast cancer. Overweight is a major risk factor for breast cancer, and high alcohol intake also increases risk. Some research appears to show high intake of plant estrogens can reduce risk, while others show increased risk. The UK's COT report on phytoestrogens concluded there is some evidence for their beneficial effects on both breast and prostate cancer based upon animal experiments, while the FSA's advice is that people at high risk of breast or prostate cancer should NOT eat a diet high in phytoestrogens. Confusing or what?

More research on humans has to be done and, meanwhile, it is probably wise to eat an overall balanced, healthy diet, such as the Menopause Eating Plan overleaf, with medium intakes of the estrogenic plant foods unless you have been specifically advised otherwise. If you think you might be at high risk of breast cancer (if one or more of your family has had it), talk to your doctor.

menopausal symptoms

Hot flashes Probably the worst symptom for many, no one knows exactly what causes them, but they can be minimized or made worse by diet.

AVOID drinking very hot drinks, alcohol, high-caffeine drinks, and hot-and-spicy meals.

GO FOR a diet high in fresh fruits, veg, salads, whole grains, and legumes. This will provide an increase in plant estrogens, which appear to minimize flashes in some women, along with regular cool water or teas, vitamin B group and E supplements. Some women report reduction in flashes using red clover, agnus castus (also called the chaste tree), and/or sage supplements; others swear by evening primrose oil. Black cohosh is no longer advised by many experts as it can have unwanted side effects.

For other menopausal symptoms, see individual articles;
▶ Dry skin, page 126;
▶ Hair condition, pages 146–8;
▶ Lack of libido, page 179;
▶ Poor memory, page 203
▶ Tiredness and insomnia, pages 186–9;
▶ Mood swings and anxiety, see Mind Matters, page 199;
▶ Joint aches and pains and headaches, pages 190–91

What are phytoestrogens? They are compounds found in many plants that have an estrogenlike effect in the body. They can be divided into flavonoids and nonflavonoids. The flavonoids are subdivided into isoflavones, such as genistein and daidzein (found mainly in legumes such as soybeans, chickpeas, and lentils), and coumestans, such as coumestrol (found mainly in sprouted legumes). The nonflavonoids are lignans, found in seeds, whole grains, and fresh fruits and vegetables.

top 10 menopause managers

brazil nuts High in selenium, which can improve the condition of dry skin and hair, increase the action of the thyroid gland, and help protect against heart disease. Other nuts are also useful sources.

fish Oily fish, such as salmon and mackerel, is high in omega-3 fatty acids to help minimize joint pain, risk of heart disease, and some cancers, and improve skin and hair condition. Shellfish is high in zinc, might help to increase libido, and is a powerful antioxidant.

3 low-fat dairy produce Contains calcium for healthy bones, heart, and nerves, which is better absorbed when high amounts of saturated fat aren't present, but small amounts of omega-3 or -6 fats are.

4 flax seeds (linseeds) High in phytoestrogens called lignans, these might reduce hot flashes, might block cancer cells in certain conditions, and are one of the few nonfish sources of omega-3s, which have a host of benefits.

5 whole grains Whole grains, such as barley, rye, and oats, contain lignans (see Flax seeds above) and other types of phytochemicals that can help protect you from heart disease and cancers.

6 spices Ginger is the most useful spice for helping to alleviate headaches and bloating; turmeric is another spice which can help minimize painful joint and other aches and pains of the menopause.

7 herbal remedies St.-John's-Wort can ease depression, a common side effect of the menopause, while gingko biloba might help your memory, and agnus castus , also known as Monk's Pepper and chaste tree, can help relieve hot flashes.

8 supplements Evening primrose oil is rich in the longer-chain omega-6 fatty acids, and some women report good results (which are not quick to kick in, nevertheless) using a daily supplement for menopausal symptoms. Vitamins B_6 and calcium supplements have been shown to improve mood and sleep in some women.

9 tofu, soy, and legumes Rich in plant estrogens called isoflavones (of which there are many sub-divisions, including genistein and daidzein), which can help to prevent heart disease, lower blood cholesterol, might help to prevent breast cancer, and are said to help alleviate hot flashes and other menopausal symptoms. If you like baking, use soy flour or at least partially replace wheat flour.

10 bean sprouts Alfalfa and mung bean sprouts are rich in coumestans, another type of natural plant estrogen. Chinese herbalists use alfalfa sprouts for menopausal symptoms.

menopause eating plan

The 7-day eating plan shown here should help to reduce menopause symptoms, such as hot flashes, sweats, tiredness, and aches and pains. The diet contains a moderately high amount of natural plant estrogens, so if you are at risk of breast cancer or actually have breast cancer, you should seek advice from your doctor before embarking on the plan.

instructions

- Follow the plan as laid out, having portion sizes to suit your appetite, unless you are overweight, in which case try to have moderate portions only.

- Eat your between-meal snacks, as eating little and often might produce fewer hot flashes than eating one big meal less frequently.

- Have about 8 glasses of water a day, or iced black tea can be used to replace 3 or 4 of these glasses.

- Take any herbal or vitamin supplements you are trying with water or along with a meal or snack.

breakfast every day

should be one of the following options:
1 A bowlful of good-quality muesli with oat flakes, rye flakes, nuts, seeds, and dried fruits, with a selection of fresh fruit of your choice chopped or sprinkled in, with 4 teaspoons flax seeds, and covered with calcium-enriched soymilk.
2 A bowl of calcium-enriched soy yogurt, 3 to 4 tablespoons fruit compote (such as apple, plum, or mixed reconstituted dried fruit), sprinkled with muesli as above and topped with flax seeds.
NOTE: Skim milk and low-fat yogurt with live bacteria can be substituted for the soymilk if you prefer, or do this every other day.

snacks

Every day have TWO between-meal snacks consisting of one of the following —try to vary your choices as much as possible:
- 5 Brazil nuts or 8 almonds
- 4 teaspoons sunflower seeds or pumpkin seeds
- 1 tablespoon good-quality hummus on 1 dark rye crispbread
- 4 teaspoons tahini on 1 organic brown rice cake
- 4 pieces (¾ cup) organic dried apricot or 2 dried figs
- fruit-flavored calcium-enriched fruit soy yogurt

day 1

lunch

Brown basmati rice and chickpea salad with your choice of chopped salad vegetables and fresh herbs added, dressed in olive oil Italian dressing

¾ cup low-fat fromage blanc or soy yogurt with honey and 1 teaspoon sunflower seeds

evening

Broiled herring fillets
Orange and Belgium endive salad
Broccoli
Rye bread with low-fat spread

day 2

lunch

Sandwich on 2 slices dark rye bread filled with ripe avocado and slices of half-fat mozzarella cheese, plus lettuce and tomatoes

Apple or peach

evening

Casserole of Scotch barley, mixed root vegetables, and tofu
Stir-fried spring greens
10 almonds

day 3

lunch

Tomato and basil soup
Soft goat cheese
3 Scottish oatcakes
1 orange or kiwi fruit

evening

Casserole of Scotch barley, mixed root vegetables, and tofu
Stir-fried spring greens
10 almonds

day 4

lunch

Whole-wheat pita bread filled with hummus and mixed salad
1 piece fruit of choice

evening

Broiled or poached salmon steak
4 teaspoons homemade pesto sauce
Green lentils
Stir-fried red bell peppers in olive oil

day 5

lunch

Feta cheese
Dark rye crispbreads
Side salad of walnuts, celery, and apple dressed with olive oil Italian dressing

evening

1 pack mixed frozen seafood, thawed and stir-fried in olive oil before tossing with 2 to 3 tablespoons good-quality tomato and basil pasta sauce before reheating; serve on brown basmati rice
Broccoli
1 piece fruit of choice

day 6

lunch

Sandwich on 2 slices dark rye bread filled with organic sugar-free peanut butter, arugula, and other salad leaves of choice
Cherry tomato and scallion salad
5 Brazil nuts

evening

Small lean beef steak, broiled
New potatoes
Green beans
Spinach

day 7

lunch

Salad of fresh bean sprouts, grated carrot, green beans, and corn kernels, dressed in olive oil Italian dressing into which you have beaten a little silken tofu
1 slice of dark rye bread
5 almonds

evening

Chicken, tomato, and thyme casserole
Brown basmati rice or quinoa
Steamed greens or spinach
Peas

body for your newlife

If you want to feel good—if you want to grab life by the tails—you need your body to be in good working order. The most simple key to achieving this is to do regular exercise, and yet 75 percent of people aged 50 and over don't do any real exercise at all.

There is a wealth of scientific research to show that keeping active and keeping fit are among the very best ways to stay in good health as we get older. In Chapter 2, we will be examining all the links between exercise, feeling good, and health protection, and showing you how best to use exercise to enhance your life.

Around the ages of 50 and 60, many people feel it's too late to begin getting more active, but that is not true. Your body is amazingly adept at coping with new demands on it—as long as you are sensible—and studies show that older bodies make improvements in fitness and appearance just as rapidly as younger ones.

If food is your body's fuel, then exercise is the catalyst that keeps you running smoothly, efficiently, and without problems … for the rest of your life.

use it or lose it! That could be the mantra for your body's health. We look at all the ways in which exercise can help us feel great.

If you're in any doubt that you can benefit from regular activity, try the body questionnaire on the following pages. You only need to do a few simple exercises, taking a few minutes of your time, then add up your score to find out how old your body really is. Most of us over 40 will probably be shocked to find that whatever the calendar says, our real age is older. The older you are in "real" terms, the more your body is crying out for exercise.

For a healthy heart, do regular exercise. So much research has now been done to prove this link beyond doubt. Indeed, an eight-year study of 22,000 men in the United States found fitness was of greater importance in maintaining heart health than being slim, so if you are fat but fit you'll live longer than if you're slim but unfit. Most studies show daily walking can reduce risk of heart disease by up to 50 percent. Similar results have been shown in beating stroke and high blood pressure, and in improving blood fat and cholesterol profiles.

Studies also link inactivity with increased risk of type-2 diabetes and some cancers. For example, exercise cuts the risk of bowel cancer by a third.

Among the most obvious signs of aging are a thickening waist, a pot belly, poor posture, and lumps and bumps where before there were none. Regular exercise, however, can reverse most of these signs, if not helping you revert to exactly how you used to be, then at least making huge improvements. Improving your shape can also improve your health. Reducing your pot belly or "apple" shape, for example, can reduce your risk of heart disease.

People who do regular exercise also find it much easier to stay slim than those who don't. This is even more important if you have dieted to lose weight. An American study of slimmers five years on from dieting found that the 70 percent who had kept all or most of their weight off had taken part in regular activities throughout that time. All the available evidence says that the weight will return unless you are active.

If you feel tired you take a rest, but there is a lot of evidence to show that the best way to feel better and more energized is to do the reverse … go out for a walk or do other light aerobic exercise, such as swimming. Exercise increases the blood flow to the brain and releases hormones that help you to feel better, as well as increasing brain power and lifting depression.

If you have a moderate backache or arthritis, tense shoulders, or unspecified aches and pains—again, rather than rest, research shows you should exercise. This will loosen up ligaments and joints, strengthen the muscles that support the bone structure, and benefit your body in several other ways.

Moreover, regular weight-bearing activity can increase bone density and minimize the risk of osteoporosis and fractures.

Even if you have trouble relaxing or getting to sleep, if you suffer from insomnia or stress, all forms of exercise will help you to relax. Activity literally releases the tension in your body, as well as sending calming hormones where they need to be.

In the pages that follow you'll find what type of exercise to do to beat your own particular problems. I hope to prove exercising can be fun—and safe, whatever your age or fitness level.

how old is your body?

Your age in years might be 40, 50, or 60—but how old is your body? Take the tests on these pages and find out whether you're really a toned 20 year old or a sagging 70. However young at heart you are, without a reasonably fit body you aren't going to feel as young as you can. The 10 tests here are easy and quick to do and the results will give you a good estimate of your true physical age.

what to do To carry out the tests wear suitable, comfortable clothing, such as a lightweight tracksuit or T-shirt and shorts, and wear trainers. Try to do the tests in a warm room when you are feeling well, not too soon after a meal.

You will need a watch with a second hand or timer, pen and paper, a measuring tape, stairs or a step platform, a flat wall that you can stand against, a ruler, and someone to help for the last test. It will be helpful if you have someone with you throughout the tests, to assess how you do, although it isn't essential.

1 stamina test— step-ups

● Stand in front of a step platform or a stair 6 to 8 inches high. Step up with the left foot, then bring up the right. Take the left foot back down, then the right. That counts as one step.
● Step up and down like this for 1 minute and count how many steps you make.

0 – 15 Add 10 years to your age
16 – 25 Add 5 years
26 – 35 Add nothing
36 – 50 Subtract 2 years
51+ Subtract 5 years

2 upper-body strength test— press-ups

● Upper-body strength and tone often get ignored. Lie on your front, placing both hands at shoulder level, but outside each one. Keeping the toes on floor and elbows below shoulder height, push into your palms to raise the upper body so your back is flat. Return your body to the floor and repeat.
● How many can you do in one minute?

0 – 15 Add 2 years
16 – 25 Add nothing
26+ Subtract 5 years

3 lower-body strength test— squats

● Stand with your feet hip-width apart, arms out in front of you, then bend knees and lower bottom as if you were going to sit down, until your thighs are parallel to the floor. Return to starting position.
● Count how many you can do in 1 minute.

0 – 15 Add 5 years
16 – 30 Add 2 years
31 – 40 Add nothing
40+ Subtract 2 years

4 abdominal strength test— sit-ups

● Lie on your back on a mat with your feet on the floor, knees bent and arms at your sides. Breathing out, slowly lift head and neck (and back if possible) off the floor and allow your arms to slide forward.
● Record how far your arms reach. Return to floor.
SAFETY NOTE: Only go as far as you are able without undue strain. If you have a bad back, don't perform this exercise, but add 5 years to your count.

Can't perform – Add 10 years
Wrists go to thighs – Add 5 years
Elbows go to thighs – Add nothing
Chest reaches thighs – Subtract 5 years

5 flexibility test 1— sit-and-reach

● Bodily stiffness, lack of flexibility in the joints, and a narrow range of movement are all associated with aging. This measures flexibility in the lower back and hamstrings, two of the first areas to stiffen with age.
● Sit on a mat with your legs straight out in front of you, hip-width apart and feet flexed, arms at your sides and lower back not slumped. Stretch out your arms toward your toes. How far can you go and HOLD for a minimum count of three? NOTE: DO NOT round out the lower back to try to reach farther.

No farther than mid-to-lower leg – Add 5 years
Around ankles – Add 2 years
To the toes, but no further – Add nothing
Beyond the toes – Subtract 3 years

6 flexibility test 2— sit-and-twist

● Spinal flexibility is important for making you able to do so many of the typical activities of youth, such as dancing and some more exotic sexual positions. Sit on a mat on the floor with back straight and legs out in front of you, feet flexed. Place right hand, palm flat, on the floor behind your lower spine and then twist shoulders around so you're looking over your right shoulder. Hold for 10 seconds.

Couldn't twist shoulders at all – Add 5 years
Could twist a little, but not enough to look over shoulder – Add 2 years
Could twist as described – Subtract 5 years

7 weight test

● Most people gain weight as they get older. How much weight have you put on since you were 25?

More than 42 pounds – Add 5 years
14 to 41 pounds – Add 2 years
Less than 14 pounds – Add nothing

8 waist circumference test

● Your waist measurement is an excellent indication of your physical condition.

Your waist measures over 40 inches if male or over 34½ inches if female? – Add 3 years
Your waist measures over 37 inches if male or over 31½ inches if female? – Add 1 year
All other measurements – Add nothing

9 posture test

Poor posture is a classic giveaway of age and can add years to the slimmest of bodies.
● Stand with your back against a wall. Can you stand with the back of your head, your shoulders, your tailbone and your heels all touching the wall at the same time?

No – Add 3 years.
Yes – Subtract 3 years

10 reflex test

Slowing reflexes are one of the main reasons older people give up competitive sports, but you can keep them sharp with regular practice. Try this test.
● Stand facing a helper with your hands extended and 6 inches apart. Get your helper to hold a ruler between your hands, with the 1-inch mark at the bottom and level with your hands, and the 12-inch mark at the top.
● Now your helper should drop the ruler and you should try to catch it immediately; repeat 6 times.
● How many times did you manage to catch the ruler before the 2-inch mark?

Not at all – Add 3 years
1–2 times – Add 2 years
3 times – Add nothing
4 times – Subtract 1 year
5 times – Subtract 2 years

working out your score

Total up all the additions and write the number here: _____

Total up all the subtractions and write the number here: _____

Take away the smallest number from the greatest and add this final total to your current age (or subtract it if your subtractions total is the larger number) to give you your true body age.
For example: you are currently aged 50, your total of additions is 20 and your total of subtractions is 12. You have 8 more additions than subtractions, so your true body age is 58.
As you work through this chapter in the months ahead, your true body age should improve.

exercise for **health**

"Enough evidence exists relating sedentary habits to poor health to classify physical inactivity as a major risk factor for early death." So say the authors of one of the most authoritative books ever on exercise, *Essentials of Exercise Physiology*. They also claim regular exercise throughout your life provides significant protection from coronary heart disease and stroke, and that people who do even mild exercise report better health than sedentary people.

Cardiovascular diseases cause approximately half of all deaths in midlifers and the elderly in the United States, and yet regular moderate exercise can reduce the risks by up to 50 percent, by reducing the heart rate, helping to reduce high blood pressure, and improving the profile of blood fats.

Exercise, it is clear, also enhances health in other ways. A cardiovascular system made fit through regular activity can also help protect us against cancer, type-2 diabetes, and obesity, while a study of 17,000 Harvard University students showed regular exercise counters the effects of cigarette smoking and excess body weight.

regular exercise Interestingly, for unfit people it takes only small improvements in the amount of exercise they do to reap important benefits. The regularity, rather than the intensity, is what counts most. Several studies show that 20 to 30 minutes walking four times a week can be enough to make a great difference in your health profile.

● A study published in the *Journal of the American Medical Association* found that women who walked for half an hour a day had a 30 percent less chance of stroke.

● A study published in the *New England Journal of Medicine* found that walking is as good as running in reducing the risk of cardiovascular disease (CVD) for women aged 50 to 79.

● And in adults with diabetes, regular walking of two hours a week lowered the death rates from all causes by 39 percent.

never too late Whether you are 40 or 60—or even 80—research shows that you can improve your fitness levels and health considerably after only a few weeks or months of exercise. One study from Texas, which monitored a group of men at age 20 and then 30 years later, found that by the age of 50 the men had become unfit and flabby —but that after a program of regular aerobic exercise their fitness profiles had returned to the same levels they had had at 20.

The consensus of professional opinion is that in midlife a healthy adult can get the aerobic capacity of a fit person 20 to 25 years younger with regular effort, however unfit at the outset.

what to do To improve your health and chances of living a long life, you simply need to do regular aerobic exercise—this is exercise which increases your heart rate. The programs overleaf will all achieve this in a total of 1 to 2 hours a week. For people of poor or moderate fitness, 90 minutes a week is plenty. Add to that a few of our suggested lifestyle changes and within three months you should see significant improvement.

the plans

On the following pages we have three simple staged exercise plans to increase your cardiovascular fitness for the benefits discussed on the previous page. Before beginning any of them, read the tips in the introduction below.

make your workout work for you

If you exercise too hard—especially if you haven't exercised much or at all in the recent past—it can be dangerous, but if on the other hand you don't push yourself hard enough, you won't improve your fitness level and gain the associated health benefits.

So it's best to aim for a very steady state of "medium-to-hard" exertion during your workout. This means that you can just about talk comfortably while you are working out. If you can't talk, you are working too hard; if you find you can chat easily, however, you are obviously not working hard enough.

For a slightly more scientific test, purchase a heart-rate monitor (these are widely available from sports equipment stores or via the Internet) and use this to make sure your heart rate is between 50 percent and 70 percent of your maximum during your workout. Maximum heart rate (MHR) equals 220 minus your age for women, or 226 minus your age for men. For example, if you are female and aged 50 your MHR is 170; 50 percent of that is 85, 60 percent is 102, while 70 percent is 119.

In the early stages of an aerobic fitness plans for older adults who haven't exercised in a while, it is best to start at the 50 percent level (in other words, keeping your heart rate at about this level throughout your workout) and then to increase this up through 60 percent and 70 percent as the weeks progress.

Before you start, and at all stages throughout, do bear in mind the safety suggestions that are listed opposite.

See also:
▶ For all cool-down stretches, see the panel on pages 82–3.

Did you know ...?

● You can buy rubbery knobbled insoles for sports shoes that absorb much more shock than standard trainers. These are ideal for people prone to knee or ankle injury and joint pain.

● You don't need an array of special supplements to help you work better when training. There is some scientific evidence to show, however, coenzyme Q10 might help unfit people work for longer.

● The US College of Sports Medicine recommends up to 2½ cups of water 2 hours before exercising and an extra ⅔ cup for each 20 minutes of aerobic exercise.

● Some research indicates if you feel very tired during or after a workout, it might not just be because you are unfit. You might be short of iron in your diet—so eat more red meat, whole grains, dark leafy greens, eggs, and dried fruit.

safety at any age

● Check with your doctor before beginning an exercise program.

● For people who are unfit or have any health problems, it is usually best to start with the walking program, but your own physician will help you decide.

● People with problems like arthritis or chronic back pain should follow an aerobic exercise program personally recommended to them by a doctor or exercise professional. This program might be suitable—show it to them and see.

● The Questionnaire on pages 64–5 will help you determine your fitness level.

● For each program, start at Level 1 and work up gradually through the levels at your own pace.

● Warm up before and cool down after each aerobic exercise session. If you don't, you can risk muscular pain and possible faintness or dizziness afterward.

● Wear good training shoes that absorb shock. Wear comfortable clothes that allow unrestricted movement for walking and cycling—tracksuit bottoms and a T-shirt are ideal.

● Monitor your exertion level while exercising (see opposite).

● Have a small snack about an hour before exercising, and don't forget to take a small water bottle with you.

● Be sensible! Start on a level that is right for you.

everyday exercises

To maximize the benefits of your structured plan, try to think of ways of increasing your activity levels in your everyday life. Research shows that you can almost double the amount of exercise you take by adopting even a few of these ideas:

● Whenever you are walking—around the mall or to the corner store—make an effort to speed up to a "training" level.

● When using your car, park a little farther away from where you want to be—most people try to park as close as possible.

● Use stairs whenever you can, and avoid elevators and escalators.

● Wear ankle weights when walking around.

● When you have waiting time, such as while cooking, use it to do some on-the-spot moves. Try marching on the spot.

● If you have music on at home, don't just sit or stand and listen—dance to it.

● If watching TV in the evening, don't sit there for hours, but get up and move around every 15 minutes or so. Use the ads to do a small chore, such as washing the dishes. If you build activity into your regular life it becomes second nature.

walking program

Warm up by walking slowly or marching on spot 3 minutes. ● Work through the levels in your own time. If you prefer, you can have Day 7 off each week, just doing three walks a week, but your progress will be slower.

	day 1	day 2	day 3	day 4	day 5	day 6	day 7
level 1	20 minutes flat walk 10 brisk* 10 moderate	●	20 minutes flat walk 10 brisk* 10 moderate	●	20 minutes flat walk 10 brisk* 10 moderate	●	20 minutes flat walk 10 brisk* 10 moderate
2	20 minutes flat walk all brisk	●	20 minutes flat walk all brisk	●	20 minutes flat walk all brisk	●	20 minutes flat walk all brisk
3	30 minutes flat walk 20 brisk 10 moderate	●	30 minutes flat walk 20 brisk 10 moderate	●	30 minutes flat walk 20 brisk 10 moderate	●	30 minutes flat walk 20 brisk 10 moderate
4	30 minutes flat walk all brisk	●	30 minutes flat walk all brisk	●	30 minutes flat walk all brisk	●	30 minutes flat walk all brisk
5	30 minutes hill walk 15 brisk 15 moderate	●	30 minutes hill walk 15 brisk 15 moderate	●	30 minutes hill walk 15 brisk 15 moderate	●	30 minutes hill walk 15 brisk 15 moderate
6	30 minutes hill walk all brisk	●	30 minutes hill walk all brisk	●	30 minutes hill walk all brisk	●	30 minutes hill walk all brisk

*Brisk is a pace that keeps your heart rate in between 50 percent and 70 percent of maximum, as explained on page 68. To improve fitness after Level 6, keep your heart rate toward the upper end, in other words near 70 percent.

cycling program

All the same as the walking program—a brisk cycling pace will keep your heart rate within the training zone—for people with low or moderate levels of fitness this will be about 8 to 12 m.p.h.; as you get fitter your speed will increase.

NOTE: Find a flat area to cycle in, as uphill work is much harder and downhill work is not aerobic.

swimming program

Strokes: Vary your strokes—such as crawl, breaststroke, backstroke, or butterfly—but always aim to swim at your best pace within your training zone for the allotted time. You can vary your strokes from day to day or within time periods.

Lengths: Until you complete Level 6, DON'T COUNT LENGTHS as this is a time- and training-zone-based program, and the amount of lengths you do will depend upon the stroke and your fitness level and strength. – JUST KEEP UP YOUR BEST PACE FOR THE TIMES GIVEN. Once you can swim for 30 continuous minutes within your training-zone heart rate, you can improve further by beginning to count lengths and do more lengths in the same time. This can be achieved by either working harder at the same stroke or changing to a harder stroke.

	day 1	day 2	day 3	day 4	day 5	day 6	day 7
level 1	20 minutes 5 x 3 minutes brisk*, plus l-minute rest between each 3-minute period**	●	20 minutes as day 1	●	20 minutes as day 1	●	●
2	25 minutes 5 x 4 minutes brisk*, plus l-minute rest between each 3-minute period**	●	25 minutes as day 1	●	25 minutes as day 1	●	●
3	30 minutes 5 x 5 minutes brisk*, plus l-minute rest between each 5-minute period**	●	30 minutes as day 1	●	30 minutes as day 1	●	●
4	33 minutes 3 x 10 minutes brisk*, plus l-minute rest between each 10-minute period**	●	33 minutes as day 1	●	33 minutes as day 1	●	●
5	33 minutes 2 x 15 minutes brisk*, plus l-minute rest between each 15-minute period**	●	33 minutes as day 1	●	33 minutes as day 1	●	●
6	30 minutes non-stop brisk swim	●	30 minutes as day 1	●	30 minutes as day 1	●	●

* Brisk is the fastest you can go while keeping within your training zone. A good test that you are maintaining this is simply that you can keep swimming continuously for the time stated—3 minutes for Level 1, 4 minutes for Level 2 , and so on. If you have to stop earlier, swim more slowly and/or use a different stroke.

** Or as long as you need to recover—but if you need more than an extra 30 to 60 seconds, you are probably swimming too fast and going outside your own training zone.

exercise for **shape**

You might have beautiful skin and no gray hair, but if your body is in bad shape no one will mistake you for someone younger. A poor shape is hard to disguise, instantly aging and revealing you've been neglecting yourself. More importantly, poor shape is linked with poor health. For example, a fat stomach can be linked with increased risk of heart disease and diabetes. However slim you are, if you don't use your body, you'll lose your shape!

So, if you don't like what you see when you look in the mirror before you get dressed in the morning, don't hurriedly turn away, put on those baggy clothes, and pretend it was someone else you glimpsed there. All those physical signs of aging in your appearance can be improved or even removed within months. A simple several-times-a-week program of exercise can re-tone your muscles, realign your body, and will smooth out, define, and appear to slim down your shape.

why work out?
When we are young, our muscles get plenty of work and have a natural tendency to keep their mass, strength, and flexibility. As we begin to age (from around the early 30s onward), however, we need to do some regular work to keep them looking good. And it is our muscle tone that most defines shape and posture—along with supple connecting tissue, which can help prevent muscle imbalance and poor posture.

Research shows that even if you have neglected your muscles and your posture for years, just a few weeks of work can show results. Within about three months, you can lose inches from your waist, redefine your arm and leg muscles, flatten your stomach, firm up your behind, ease back pain, and improve flat feet, round shoulders, and other posture problems. Even people in their 60s and beyond can improve their shape with exercise.

what to do?
The 10-exercise plan that appears on the next few pages is all that most people need to give themselves a body with the definition, tone, and shape of someone several years younger—or at least the body YOU had a few years ago!

giveaway signs of a neglected body

Thick waist As both sexes age, their waists tend to thicken, but this is a problem that particularly shows on women—partly because the waist is more defined in young women than it is in men, so the difference is more noticeable as we age, and partly because hormonal changes at the time of the menopause cause women to thicken around the middle. Regular toning and stretching exercises can minimize these effects.

Fat belly Stomach muscles don't naturally get as much exercise as other body parts (for example, leg muscles used for walking) so they tend to be the first set of muscles to show neglect. As there is nothing to hold the stomach in except muscle, a protruding stomach is a sure sign of poor stomach muscle tone.

Flat bottom Long hours sitting in chairs, cars, and so on soon show in your gluteals—muscles that once gave you a nice rounded bottom. They get elongated and flat—and your bum low-slung, flat, and flabby. A few minutes gluteal exercise daily can reverse this.

No tone to limbs This is why women of 50 stop wearing sleeveless tops and skirts above the knee (the pocket of flab just above the knee where there used to be a hollow), and men no longer parade around the pool. Unused bodies lack the undulation of strong smooth muscles. Working out with light weights or your own body weight can give you back a pleasing outline.

General bad posture Years of sitting and standing in lazy or wrong ways give many midlifers very poor posture. This shows as rounded shoulders, head poked forward, slightly flat feet, stuck-out belly, and shortened waist, and it is often combined with very poor flexibility and range of movement in the joints. Realigning exercises can improve posture tremendously, while a few lifestyle changes can make improvement permanent.

the shape program

The routine here, including warm up and cool down exercise, should not take more than 20 minutes. Do it at least three times a week—four is better—and you will see real improvement in your shape within weeks. Before you begin, read the tips below.

- Exercise in a warm room on a stable mat or towel on carpet. Wear comfortable clothes and lightweight trainers.

- Don't exercise after a heavy meal.

- Read the instructions carefully and look at the illustrations so you know what you are trying to achieve.

- Do each exercise slowly and steadily, hurrying is counterproductive.

- Breathe normally throughout, unless otherwise instructed.

- If you feel any pain, stop.

- Repeat each move up to 10 times (you might only manage fewer to start with) before resting for 20 seconds and then moving onto the next exercise.

- Don't skip the warm up—your body will perform better if it is properly warmed and there will be less risk of any muscle strain, pain, or injury.

- Don't skip the cool-down stretches. These not only help prevent stiff or sore muscles and maintain muscle elasticity, but also help prevent muscle imbalance.

- Check with your doctor before starting this or any exercise program.

warm up start of program

March on the spot for 3 minutes, starting slowly and gently and working up to a more energetic march with the arms swinging and knees lifting higher. For the last 30 seconds, circle your arms. Breathe slowly and deeply throughout.

cool down end of program

Do each leg and back stretch described in Exercise for your Weight on pages 82–3, and then add on the following six stretches:

Breathing slowly and deeply can help you to go farther into the stretch.

1 gluteal stretch Lie on your back with your knees bent and your feet flat on floor. Cross your right ankle over your left thigh near the knee and bring your legs slowly in toward your chest. Feel the stretch in the right bottom area and hip. Hold for a slow count of 10, then return to the starting position and repeat on the other side.

2 lower-back stretch From the same starting position as the gluteal stretch, bring both knees in toward your chest, clasping your hands behind your thighs. Feel the stretch in the lower back and hold for a count of 10.

3 abdominal stretch Turn over and lie on your stomach. Bend your arms with your weight on the lower arms, so your upper body is off the floor as shown. Lift your chest and look ahead of you until you feel a stretch along your abdomen. Hold for a count of 10.

4 chest stretch Sit on the floor and place your hands behind your ears, with your elbows out to your sides. Now gently pull the arms back to feel the stretch across the chest. Hold for a count of 10.

5 shoulder stretch Remain sitting on the floor and bring your right arm across your body. Use your left hand to press gently above the right elbow to bring the right arm in toward your chest, while keeping your right shoulder down. Feel the stretch in your right shoulder. Hold for a count of 10, then repeat with the left arm.

6 side stretch Remain sitting on the floor. Cross your legs and let your left arm support you to the side of your left hip. Bring your right arm up toward the ceiling and over your body until you feel the stretch up your right side. Hold for a count of 10, return to the starting position and repeat on your left side with your right arm supporting.

the shape program

1 parallel squats for the thighs, hips, and bottom

Stand with your legs shoulder-width apart, knees relaxed, hands on your waist. Pull the tummy in and tuck the bottom in, your shoulders should be back and down, but keep the posture light, not tight.

Now slowly bend the knees and hips to lower your torso toward the floor, to a maximum of 90 degrees (although you probably won't be able to go that far). Slowly return to standing.

2 lateral arm raises with weights for the shoulders

Take two 2¼-pound weights (or water-filled 750ml bottles) and stand in the starting position (see exercise 1), but with your arms at your sides. Hold your weights so your palms face in to your body. Now slowly raise your arms outward and upwards until they are at shoulder height, then slowly lower back to the starting position. Remember to keep your stomach stable while doing this exercise, and don't arch your back.

3 bicep curls with weights for the front of the upper arms

Still holding the weights, stand in the same starting position as before, but with your elbows at your waist. Have your arms in front of you and held down with the palms facing upward; grip the weights. Now slowly lift your lower arms (from hands to elbows) up and in towards your shoulders and then slowly return to start.

4

4 tricep dips for the backs of the upper arms

Sit on the floor with your legs bent and upper body slightly back, with the weight supported on your palms placed about 9 inches behind you as shown (4 left). Now bend your elbows and slowly lower your upper body down toward the floor until you are at about 45 degrees (4a above). Slowly return to the starting position.

5

5 curl-ups abdomen

Lie on the floor on your back with your knees bent, your feet flat on the floor, and your arms at your sides. There should be a small gap between your lower back and the floor, but try to keep your stomach tucked in. Lift your head off the floor and, as you do so, very slowly slide your arms toward your knees. Slowly return to the starting position.

NOTE: If this exercise hurts your neck, place a folded towel under your head or consider purchasing an abdominal exerciser cage. In later weeks you can put your hands behind your head to make the curl a little more difficult.

the shape program

6 diagonal curl-ups for the waist

Start in the same position as for the previous exercise and raise your head and neck off the floor as before, but this time move both arms across your body as if you are trying to reach a point to the side of your right knee. Slowly return to the starting position and repeat to the other side. This counts as one move.

6

7

7 double curl-ups for the abdominals

Position your legs as before, but put your hands under your neck. Slowly raise your legs into the air as shown (left), so your knees are bent and your legs are in toward your chest, then cross your ankles. Now raise your head and neck off the floor (with hands behind your head) and tilt your bottom off the floor a little as you do so (7a). Feel your abdomen working. This is a harder exercise than the previous two, so try only one or two repetitions at first and build up gradually. Slowly return to the starting position, but don't place your legs back on the floor until you have completed your reps; just move them back sufficiently to return your bottom to the floor.

7a

8 shoulder raises **for the lower back**

Turn over onto your stomach, with your legs out straight, although relaxed at the knee. Bend your arms and place your hands under your forehead as shown. Now slowly raise your upper body, head, and arms a few inches off the floor, or as far as you can comfortably go, which might be only an inch or so. Slowly return to the starting position. Always keep your legs in contact with the floor and still.

8

9

9 press-ups **for the pectorals (chest) and triceps**

Kneel on all fours with your back straight, tummy tucked in, arms under the shoulders and your fingers pointing forward. Now slowly lower your body so your forehead nearly touches the floor. Slowly return to the starting position.

10 the bridge **for the bottom**

Lie on your back with your knees bent and your feet flat on the floor, and with your arms at your sides and the palms facing down. Now lift your bottom off the floor slowly until your thighs and body form a diagonal line to the floor. Feel your gluteals working to do this, and keep yourself there for a second before returning slowly to the floor. In later weeks you can hold the position and slowly extend one leg to finish the "line," then repeat with the other leg.

10

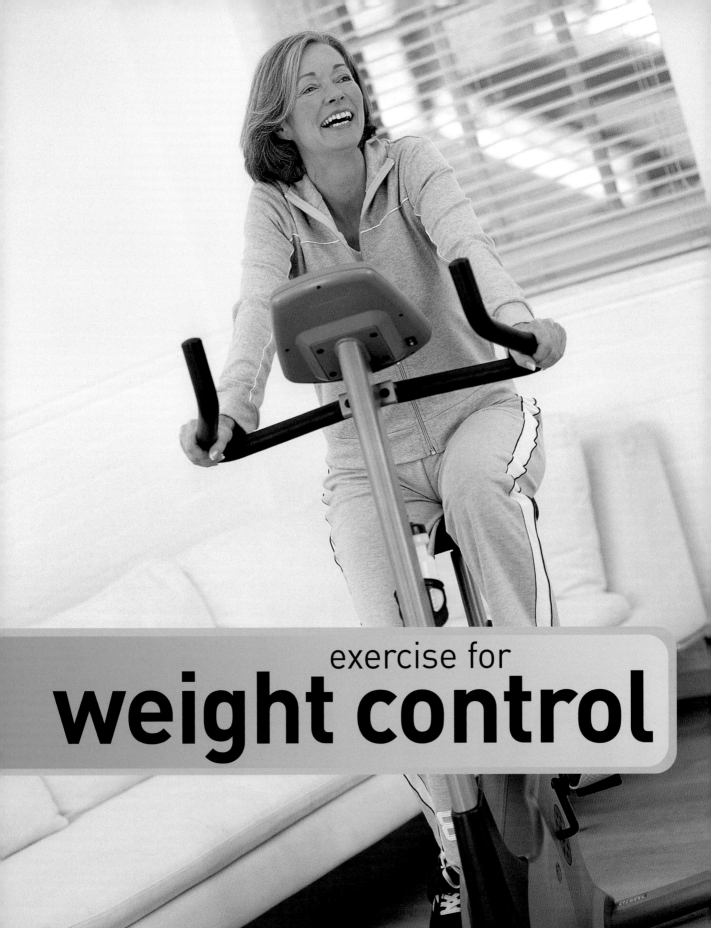

exercise for
weight control

Whether you want to lose weight or simply keep the pounds at bay, the best thing to do is to incorporate regular exercise into your life. This is a simple fact that can't be argued with, as all studies done in recent years show that it is people who keep active who find it easiest to stay slim. And in midlife exercise can be more important than at any other time of your life.

Yet, as we head into our 40s, 50s and 60s, we tend to slow down… often without realizing it. No more competitive sports; no more public transporting or walking to work as we get well off enough to commute by car or take taxis; no more cleaning —we can afford to pay someone to do it. And life often is not such a rush—so instead of going everywhere at top speed, we have more time and inclination to dawdle. Just think back to your 20s and early 30s and compare your lifestyle then with now – and I bet you find that you HAVE slowed down. That means you are using fewer calories. A hundred calories a day fewer burnt means a yearly weight gain of about 10 pounds— unless you eat 100 calories a day less to compensate.

The next part of the weight equation is that, in mid life, our natural metabolic rate (MR) begins to slow down, as a part of the general slowing down of the system which carries on until we die. This is true of both sexes, but women experience a particularly marked decline in metabolism around their late 40s and 50s—the menopausal years.

Lastly, the metabolic rate also declines on a par with our loss of muscle. The percentage of muscle (lean tissue) in your body governs, to a large extent, how high or low your metabolic rate is. The more muscle you have, the higher your basal metabolic rate will be (the rate at which you burn calories while doing no work at all, such as when you are lying down or sleeping). As we age, we tend to lose muscle steadily.

One study shows that from the ages of 30 to 70, we lose 30 percent of our lean tissue, which is one reason why younger people have higher MRs than older people. Regular exercise of the right kind can help you to not only hold onto your lean tissue, but actually reverse the loss. One study showed that using resistance (weight-training) programs, women put on 13¼ pounds of lean tissue in 20 weeks, another showed gains of 5¼ pounds over 10 weeks for men, and all the participants lost body fat as they gained lean tissue.

So what does this mean? In essence, the older you get, the more you need to counteract this metabolic slowdown by taking plenty of calorie-burning exercise (mainly aerobic) and plenty of muscle-conserving exercise (mainly weight-bearing).

Many people ask me, "Is it possible to lose weight just with exercise alone – without changing your eating habits?" The answer is that losing weight just through exercise can be very time-consuming, but it is theoretically possible for a sedentary person to lose about half a pound a week if they begin to exercise regularly. You would need to burn about 1,750 calories to lose half a pound of body fat, in other words 250 calories extra a day, which roughly translates as an hour's moderate aerobic exercise. That is a simple equation, as it doesn't take account of any increase in your metabolic rate through increasing your lean tissue or making your overall lifestyle more active.

Studies show the best results are achieved with a program that combines moderate calorie reduction with regular exercise. Once the slimming is over, however, and you just want to maintain weight—then exercise IS definitely your answer. Keep active and you'll keep the surplus pounds off for good.

burning the calories

If you need to lose weight, aim for a minimum of 5 to 6 exercise sessions a week of sufficient duration that you burn at least 250 calories a session. If you are unfit, however, build up to this level gradually. I suggest you start with any of the programs—walking, cycling, or swimming on pages 70–71. Once you have reached Level 6 on one of those programs, increase the number and duration of the sessions. If you need to maintain weight, 3 to 4 sessions a week burning at least 200 calories, should be enough to keep the pounds at bay.

The chart on page 85 shows 30 different ways to burn up 100 and 250 calories, and each activity is star-rated for its lean-tissue-building ability. Before starting any of the activities, check with your doctor that they are suitable for you—particularly if you haven't exercised in some time or have health problems.

In the long term, you should find activities you enjoy and fit in with your life, otherwise you won't stick to any plan. Below are some of my favorite suggestions for aerobic exercise you might consider. Don't forget to warm up before you begin, cool down in a similar way, and do the cool-down stretches opposite (adding those for the back if you have been swimming). More detailed safety (and other) tips for aerobic exercise appear on page 69.

aerobic exercise

skipping If you are short of time, skipping is one of the best calorie-burning activities. Indeed, unless you are quite fit, to begin with you will find it difficult to skip for longer than a minute or two. Do one or two mini-sessions a day (stopping for a few seconds now and then) until you can do several minutes without stopping. As you get more proficient, skip faster or do double jumps (jump twice in the time the rope turns), or try squatting jumps or high knee lifts. (You can buy a jump rope with a built-in calorie-counter.) You must wear good training shoes with maximum shock-absorption capacity.

dancing Whether you choose to buy a dance exercise video and prance in front of the TV, go to a dance exercise class, or actually go out dancing, exercise to music is one of the activities that is most fun to do. The music helps motivate you and is also very good for your mood, lifting depression and—according to research at Brunel University, in London—it can even help you to get fit more quickly by encouraging you to keep going longer and work a bit harder. If you are unfit, choose a beginners' video or class, and progress to fast and furious disco or hip-hop tracks.

"spinning" Much more than just riding an exercise bike at the gym, "spinning" classes are popular throughout the world now and particularly popular with men. You go for a "spin" on a stationary mountain bike and can climb steep hills or pedal flat out on the flat. The spin teacher encourages you and you "spin" to loud techno music. A 60-minute "spin" class can burn off more calories than almost any other activity.

1 standing hamstring stretch

Stand with your legs together, then slide the right foot forward and bend your left knee, leaning your body forward and resting your hands on your left thigh as shown. Lean forward from the hips and lift your bottom up, until you feel the stretch up the back of your right thigh. Repeat to the other side.

2 standing lower-calf stretch

Stand with your knees slightly bent and your right leg set a few inches behind your left leg as shown. Bend the right knee a little, keeping the heel of the right foot flat on the floor. Feel the stretch in the lower right calf as you do this. Repeat to the other side.

3 standing quad stretch

Stand with your knees relaxed and lift your right leg behind your body as shown, grasping the foot firmly with your right hand. Support yourself with a sturdy chair back if you like. Bring the foot in toward your bottom, keeping your pelvis steady. Feel the stretch up the front of your right thigh. Repeat to the other side.

cool-down stretches hold each stretch for a count of 15

4 **standing back stretch**

Stand with your feet hip width apart, knees bent, and your palms flat on your thighs, fingers facing inward. Now curve your spine and stretch out your back as shown, feeling your abdomen pulling inward as you do so.

5 **upper-calf stretch**

With the right leg, take a step back about 18 inches and bend your left leg at the knee over your shoe-laces. Keeping the heel on the floor, straighten your right leg and now lean forward slightly and feel a stretch in the upper right calf. Repeat to the other side.

▶ Invest in a pedometer (about $10—20), which will tell you how many steps you take in a day. For weight loss, aim for 10,000 steps a day; for weight control, 5,000 steps a day.

tips for resistance exercise

- If doing resistance training without professional help, carefully follow the instructions that come with your equipment.

- Start off carefully and build up gradually. For free weights, do one set of 8 to 10 reps for each of the exercises, which should come with the equipment, with a light weight to begin, for example, and then increase the sets and/or reps and/or weight lifted over time.

- Train every other day, or—when you are much stronger—do upper body work one day and lower body work the next day.

- Fewer reps using higher resistance build more lean tissue. More reps using lower resistance are better for toning and endurance.

- Warm up and cool down as for cardiovascular exercise.

- Exercise in a warm room.

- Try to build more resistance work into your everyday life – e.g. carrying shopping bags rather than pushing trolleys.

resistance work

Increasing the percentage of lean tissue (muscle) in your body through resistance exercise is, as we've seen, one of the two major ways of increasing metabolic rate and thus burning calories. Not only that, but resistance work—essentially, working with weights—also helps improve your shape, increases bone density, and—looking to the future—will help you retain physical fitness into old age. One research study found that older people who did resistance training found everyday living easier and even walked faster.

As you can see from the Activity Chart opposite, not that many activities actually increase lean tissue by any great amount. Here we look at the ways to get resistance work into your life—one is bound to be right for you.

gym work Today's health clubs and gyms usually offer state-of-the-art variable weight-resistance machines which, when properly used, are very safe and suitable for anyone from beginners onward. Reputable clubs will make sure you have a resistance program suitable for your fitness, health, and ability, and will give you a fitness assessment and induction before you begin. If you have any health problems, they should also ask for a letter from your doctor.
Pros Top-quality equipment, monitoring, motivation.
Cons Can be expensive, although community gyms are not. If you have to travel miles, you might not go as often as you should.

home gym An alternative, which might work out less expensive eventually than health club fees, is to buy equipment for your own home, such as an all-in-one multigym or minigym. These can vary in price from several hundred dollars to tens of thousands.
Pros Your are more likely to work out if you don't have to go far.
Cons No one to help you, so the equipment can gather dust unless you are motivated; space needed.

free weights With a set of dumbbells, a barbell, and various weights from 1 pound up to 10 pounds, you can perform a wide range of lean-tissue-building exercises at home.
Pros Inexpensive; can do at home.
Cons No one to help you; free weights may be dangerous if not used correctly; space needed if using bench.

other small equipment You can buy resistance bands or tubes of different resistance strengths, and achieve similar results to light weights.
Pros Inexpensive, portable (ideal for traveling), little storage space needed.
Cons As you get stronger, this equipment might not offer enough resistance.

body weight If you are very unfit, you can build a certain amount of lean tissue using your body's own weight for resistance. For example, the toning exercises in Exercise for Shape, pages 72—9, can offer a marginal increase in lean tissue.
Pros No equipment needed.
Cons Not as effective as other methods for lean-tissue building.

choosing your activity

NOTE: Always choose an activity that is suitable for your current fitness level. Activities are listed in order of fastest to slowest calorie-burners and figures are approximate. The heavier you are, the more calories you will burn doing the activity. These figures are based on a person weighing 147 pounds.
● little or no lean-tissue building; ●● builds lean tissue in legs over time, depending on intensity; ●●● good lean-tissue building; ●●●● excellent lean-tissue building.

activity	to burn 100 calories (minutes)	to burn 250 calories (minutes)	lean tissue rating (see above)
squash	7	17.5	●●
spinning	7.3	18.3	●
skipping	9	22.5	●●
stair climbing (or stair machine)	10	25	●●●
swimming, crawl	11	27.5	●
core training	11.2	28	●
circuit training (gym)	12	30	●●●●
jogging	12.5	31.3	●●
kickboxing	13	32.5	●
swimming, breast stroke	13	32.5	●
uphill walking	13	32.5	●●
ashtanga yoga	13.7	34.3	●
horse-riding	14	35	●
tennis	14	35	●
rowing (or machine)	14	35	●●●
badminton	15	37.5	●
cycling, fast	15	37.5	●●
dancing, disco or line	15	37.5	●
digging, heavy	15	37.5	●●
downhill skiing	15	37.5	●
mowing, push-type	15	37.5	●
aerobics class	16	40	●
walking, brisk	16	40	●
golf, average	20	50	●
rollerblading	20	50	●
weight training	21	52.5	●●●●
table tennis	22	55	●
cycling, moderate to slow	25	62.5	●
housework, average	25	62.5	●
lawn bowls	33	82.5	●
dancing, ballroom	33	82.5	●

exercise for **energy**

If you are one of those people who equates exercise with tiredness, fatigue, and the urgent need to lie down, you'll be wondering how it can actually energize you. Tackled in the right way, however, indeed it can. Exercise can sometimes be better than sleep for helping you to feel fresh and lively. It can be a big boost for both mental and physical energy, and can help revamp your sex life and your sleep patterns.

To be energizing, exercise doesn't always have to be energetic—although sometimes it can be. Here are the ways in which exercise energizes.

banishing tiredness
Exercise—particularly aerobic exercise, which gets the heart beating faster and the lungs breathing in more deeply, speeds the circulation of blood around the body and delivers more oxygen to the brain and muscles — indeed, to all parts of the body. This has the effect of revitalization and is especially good at alleviating "brain tiredness" or feelings of tiredness that seem to come on for little reason during the day, or after a carbohydrate meal. Exercising outdoors, in cool air, also has a refreshing and revitalizing effect.

increasing alertness and mental energy
Research shows regular exercise improves mental stamina and energy. It might do this by increasing the amount of blood and oxygen—and therefore nutrients—that reaches the brain. Exercise speeds up the metabolic rate and appears to increase brain activity—speeding up thought processes and giving you a sharpness that shows in faster speech and more lucid expression. Because exercise lifts depression, it can clear the mental "fog" that makes depressed people seem slow to react. Canadian research shows that depressed people improve with as little as 20 minutes' exercise three times a week. Exercise makes us breathe more deeply, which in turn calms us and helps us feel more self-confident, improving performance.

increasing strength
Resistance exercise (see pages 84–5) helps strengthen and build lean tissue. Increased strength means you can work longer, and harder, at all physical activities and this can help to prevent physical tiredness.

reviving sexual energy
Improved circulation and strength can help revive libido and improve sexual performance. One cause of impotence in males is a diminished blood supply to the penis, for example. And female sexual sensitivity is enhanced with improved blood supply to the vaginal area.

improving quality of sleep
If you exercise regularly, research shows your quality of sleep improves — you sleep more deeply, more soundly, and wake more refreshed.

stimulating hormones
Exercise can release hormones, such as dopamine and serotonin, which can lift depression, banish the feelings of lethargy and fatigue that depression often brings, and produce a sense of well-being sometimes known as the "exercise high."

don't overexercise Doing too much, too soon, or overtaxing your muscles or heart and lungs WILL make you feel tired. The best exercise for energy is moderate and is something you enjoy.

don't exercise when you are genuinely tired For example, if you have been up for 18 consecutive hours without sleep, it will be better to go to bed than start exercising to try to find energy.

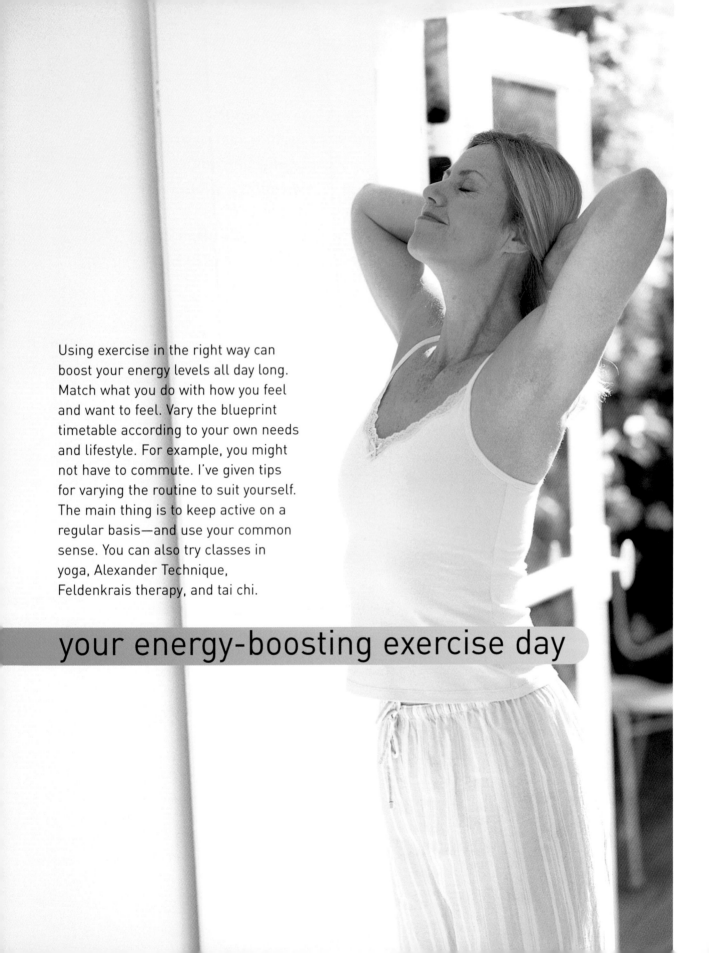

Using exercise in the right way can boost your energy levels all day long. Match what you do with how you feel and want to feel. Vary the blueprint timetable according to your own needs and lifestyle. For example, you might not have to commute. I've given tips for varying the routine to suit yourself. The main thing is to keep active on a regular basis—and use your common sense. You can also try classes in yoga, Alexander Technique, Feldenkrais therapy, and tai chi.

your energy-boosting exercise day

7 a.m.—on waking

If you've slept with an open window you shouldn't feel too sluggish—but now is a good time to go over to that window and do some deep breathing to get oxygen circulating around your body. Couple it with some shoulder shrugs and small arm circles, and within a minute or two you should feel wide awake.

Any stiffness from the night? Arch your back (see warm-up exercises on page 74) and slowly and gently bring your head down first to your right shoulder and then up and over to your left, looking forward all the time.

8.30 a.m.—journey to work

After a small healthy breakfast, if possible build some exercise into your morning commute. Even if you can't walk or cycle all the way, perhaps you can walk to the next bus or train stop instead of the nearest one, or get off at a stop farther away from work. If you drive in to work, could you park a bit farther away?

Even 15 minutes' walking in the morning will get your heart rate up, improve your circulation, help burn off calories, and will boost brain power so you work better. If you have any stress about work, the walk will also help you to relax.

tips ● If you don't commute, build in a never-to-be-missed 15 to 30 minutes to get out of your home and bring your body to life with some exercise. ● Don't try to do hard aerobic or resistance work too early in the morning—most people's bodies can't cope at this time; wait until early evening if possible.

11.30 a.m.—break time

After a few hours at work, you might be feeling stressed out mentally, as morning is when most pressure is on. Use a 10-minute break to have a change of scene—walk up a few flights to take in a view from the roof terrace; walk down to the grounds, or, if that isn't possible, do some stretches in the stockroom or boardroom. No one should go more than 2 to 3 hours sitting or standing in the same place without a break. A banana and a cup of tea make ideal break-time snack food.

tip ● If you are at home, you too should take a break from whatever you're doing. A few minutes on a rebounder would be a good pick-you-up.

1.30 p.m.—lunch

Take at least a 20-minute walk before your lunch and incorporate some deep breathing (see pages 110–11). Make lunch high in protein and low in carbs, so you don't suffer a slump in the afternoon.

tip ● If your schedule means you have to go to the gym or a class in your lunch break, skip workout time later.

3 p.m.—afternoon break

By now you might be feeling a bit stiff around the shoulders, neck, or lower back and generally a bit tired or tense, especially if you work at a desk or do a lot of driving or standing for long hours. You need to do five minutes' stretching to suit your own problem areas (see stretches on pages 82–3). Relax your face with some forced yawns and cup your hands over your eyes to ease eye strain. A green tea and an apple will complete your quick afternoon re-energizer.

6.30 p.m.—workout time

Research shows about 6 to 7p.m. is the best time to ask your body to do formal exercise—such as gym work, an exercise class, or a workout video in front of the TV. So rather than rushing home to a cocktail, use the gym as your tonic! If you're planning to do the workouts in this book, now is the time. Follow them with an invigorating shower before supper. Don't leave aerobic or resistance training any later than 8p.m., otherwise you might not sleep well.

tip ● If your working hours carry on until 7p.m. or so, try to do your workout before you commute home.

10 p.m.—winding down

Now you need wind-down exercise to help you sleep well. Yoga and/or stretching are ideal, but you don't need to do more than 10 to 15 minutes.

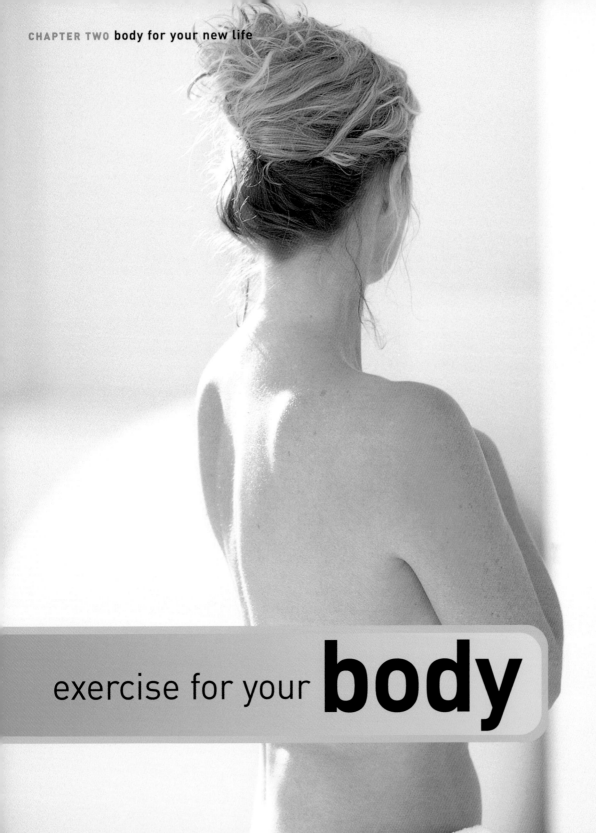

exercise for your **body**

As we move out of young adulthood into so-called "middle age," one of the most shocking things that can happen to us—worse even than the first sighting of a wrinkle or gray hair—is the realization that we have "aches and pains." For years we sail through life mistreating our bodies and taking them for granted and now, suddenly—or so it seems—the body is paying us back... back pain, joint pain, neck pain, hip pain, knee pain ...

Even if there isn't a lot of pain as such, we can find we can't reach or stretch or twist or run quite as well as we used to. Or that there is a certain stiffness in the back or hips after a few hours in bed, or that joints sprain more easily than they used to.

The fact is that a sedentary lifestyle causes—or makes worse—most of these complaints and symptoms, and that regular activity can keep almost any body in good working order and largely free from the disabilities that signal the end of youth. But it is never too late to reverse these symptoms. In one American study residents of a nursing home with an average age of 87, just 10 weeks' training of 2$\frac{1}{4}$ hours a week improved their strength, fitness, gait, balance, and speed by up to 100 percent.

In the next few pages, we look at how exercise can minimize back, joint, and muscular aches and pains, and help to prevent the bone degeneration that can lead to osteoporosis.

back pain
Back pain is a world-wide problem. The American college of Rheumatology estimates two-thirds of all adults experience at least one episode of back pain during their lifetime. The college also estimates low back pain disables 5.4 million Americans, and costs at least $16 billion each year. And yet many back problems are preventable if we do some simple daily exercises and keep active, and most bad backs can be "cured" with similarly simple remedial exercises.

arthritis and stiff joints
It is now believed that osteoarthritis pain can be minimized with exercise, and age-associated stiffness is often a result of inactivity and inflexibility in the joints.

rheumatism and fibromyalgia
According to scientific research, muscular aches and random pains might be sporadic, acute, or chronic, and are often included under the umbrella of rheumatism or fibromyalgia, can be significantly improved with regular exercise.

osteoporosis
The loss of bone density which can lead to osteoporosis can be minimized with regular exercise. Although bone loss doesn't cause pain in its initial stages, and can be hard to detect without a scan, in later middle age and old age it can cause fractures, skeletal shrinking and misalignment, and considerable incapacity—so it is well worth beginning a bone maintenance program as soon as possible.

exercises for your back

The routine here, including warm-up and cool-down, should take you no more than 20 minutes. Do it at least three times a week—four is even better—and you will see real improvement in your shape within weeks. Before you begin, however, read all the tips below.

In recent years there has been a big change in the way experts suggest we manage back pain. Bed rest used to be prescribed, but staying in bed for days usually serves only to weaken the muscles that support the back even farther, and stiffens the whole body. In most cases, this only makes your back worse, while keeping active and following the right kind of exercise plan can reduce pain and increase mobility.

Most acute back pain is caused when a muscle or ligament is pulled via sudden overuse—very common in midlife, as we tend to use our backs only infrequently, which makes them weak, and then do something like very heavy lifting or digging, or even just twisting into an unusual position, such as when reaching for something.

Then there is "wear-and-tear" back pain, caused by the disks in the spine becoming less flexible, thinner, and less able to absorb shock. This can cause the vertebrae to move closer together, and this in turn causes pain and strain. Also you can have a "slipped disc," when one or more discs press on the nerves that run along the length of the spine, which also causes pain. Adequate fluid and fatty-acid intake (see Chapter 1) and regular exercise to preserve back and abdominal muscles will help prevent the pain of "wear and tear" by offering support and stability; stretching exercises help maintain back flexibility, which is often very poor in older adults, and also help to release muscle tension, which can cause chronic long-term back pain. Exercise can also maintain bone density, which helps preserve the spine and prevent pain.

For what to do during an acute attack of back pain, see opposite. For maintaining your back in good condition, and thus helping prevent recurring back pain, try the exercises on the following pages.

look at your lifestyle

To help prevent or minimize back pain, use the following tips in everyday life:

- When carrying, try to distribute weight evenly in both hands.

- When lifting, bend at the knees, keep your abdominals tight, and your feet wide apart, and lift the object keeping it as close to your body as you can.

- When sitting, don't slump in the chair. Try to use chairs that have a depth that matches your upper leg length, as well as a supportive back.

- Use a good mattress—medium-firm suits most people— and use only one pillow.

- Evidence suggests that there is an emotional component with much back pain.

- Anxiety, depression, and stress can all make pain worse. Research reported in the *Journal of Industrial Medicine* found that people who are unhappy at work or who have to work at pressure are more likely to feel back pain than other people.

helpful tools for a bad back

- A wooden backstretcher (widely available) which you lie on, on the floor, can help improve posture and posture-related back problems.

- Chiropractors and osteopaths are recognized as being able to help maintain a healthy back by manipulation and massage. They are excellent for restoring an acute back to the nonpainful stage.

- Deep-tissue massage (Swedish, physio-therapy) can relieve back pain by aiding relaxation.

- Acupuncture can help acute back pain where other methods have failed or can't be used.

acute back pain

- First apply to the painful area an ice pack or frozen peas covered with a towel. This helps reduce inflammation.

- Then apply warmth, such as a hot-water bottle, to the surrounding area. It will help the surrounding muscles, which might have gone into spasm to try to protect the area, to relax.

- Painkillers taken in the first 24 hours of bad back pain will also help the muscles to come out of spasm, and, therefore, get you out of the common spiral when you feel pain and tense up even more because of it.

- Rest on your back for a few hours if necessary and, while you do so, try exercises 1 and 2 on the following page regularly to ease the pain.

- When the pain moves from "pain" to the lesser category of "ache," begin exercises 3 and 4 on page 95 and try to move around as much as you can, without twisting or sudden movements.

- See your doctor for advice if your back pain is no better in 24 hours—and if it was caused by a fall or other obvious injury, if you have trouble passing urine, if you have pain or numbness in your legs, or the pain worsens.

- Do regular back exercises (exercises 5 to 9 on the following pages, the stretches on pages 75 and 82–3, and the abdominal exercises on pages 77–8). Keep active to prevent future attacks.

- The exercises for your joints, bones, and relaxation are also relevant (see pages 98–107 and 112–13).

exercises for your back

2 the rock

Start from the same position as exercise 1, but, as you bring your knees in to your chest, lift your neck slightly and rock slowly back and forth, massaging your spine with the movement. NOTE: This is for lower-back pain—if you have neck pain, stick to exercise 1.

1 the pull-in

Lie on your back (on a comfortable floor mat or your bed) with your knees bent in toward your chest. Clasp your knees just below the joint around the front, as shown, and relax. Now gently pull both knees in farther toward your chest and feel the stretch in your lower back. Relax and repeat several times, several times a day.

4 back arch

Kneel on all fours on a floor mat with your hands shoulder-width apart. Look down at the floor as you arch your back, breathing out and pulling your stomach in as you do so. Now slowly lower your stomach toward the floor, breathing in and hollowing your back slightly, and look up to the ceiling.

5 walking hands

Kneel on all fours on a floor mat with your hands shoulder-width apart. Now, without any sudden twisting movements, slowly "walk" your hands around to the right side as far as you can without undue strain. Slowly walk them back to middle and then around to the left side. Repeat 10 times.

3 hip rotation

Lie on your back on a comfortable floor mat or your bed, with your knees bent and your feet flat on the floor or bed. Now lift your right foot from the floor and in a few inches toward your chest, clasping your hand around the knee as in exercise 1. Keeping your left foot firmly on the floor or bed and your left leg still, gently rotate the right knee clockwise to rotate the right hip. Do this 10 times, then rotate counterclockwise, and repeat with the left leg.

exercise for your back

6 raising hands

Start as in exercise 5. Balancing carefully on your left hand, lift your right hand from the floor and reach under your body toward your lower abdomen (left), then slowly and in a controlled way, swing the arm out to your right side (with the arm straight but loose at the elbow), following the movement with your eyes, and return it to starting position (6a and b). Repeat with the left hand.

7 knee rises

Start as in exercise 6. Now, balancing carefully on your left knee, lift your right knee up and aim to touch your left elbow—just going as far as you can without undue strain. Return to the starting position and repeat up to 10 times, then repeat with your left knee.

8 lying raises

Lie on an exercise mat or towel on the floor with your face down and hands on each side of head. Now, breathing in, gently try to raise your head and legs a few inches off the floor, and hold for up to 20 seconds. Breathe out and gently return to floor, and repeat up to 10 times.

9 lying hip and bottom stretch

Lie on the floor on your back with your knees bent and feet flat on the floor, hip-width apart. Now bring your right foot off the floor and in to rest on the top of the left thigh near the knee. Then move your left leg slowly down to the side so your left knee touches the floor (or as near as you can get without undue strain), as shown. As you go, you will feel a stretch across your right hip and bottom— the more the feel of the stretch, the tighter your bottom and hips are. This is a common cause of low back pain. Hold for a count of up to 20, then return to the starting position and repeat to the other side.

other exercise to

pilates Concentrates on improving abdominal strength and flexibility to improve posture and back strength.

alexander technique Helps improve posture and relaxation, and helps the back to work with minimum strain on the spine.

gyrotonics Similar to pilates, but with more emphasis on three-dimensional movement. This might be ideal for back maintenance, rather than beginner's work.

yoga Improves flexibility, posture, and relaxation, and might improve strength, too. (See pages 112–13 for more on yoga.)

exercises for your joints

If your joints are painful or stiff, or ache from time to time, you need to do regular flexibility work. Arthritis can also be helped with gentle exercise. If you have rheumatoid arthritis, it is best to rest when you have a flare-up and exercise at other times. Research shows the best treatment for osteoarthritis is not to avoid exercise, as many do, but to keep as active as you can. And, if you have muscular aches and pains (often called "fibromyalgia" if severe), you will benefit from keeping active (see below). For anyone with stiffness and/or muscular aches or pains, it will help if you have a warm bath before exercise, if you take regular omega-3 fish oils, and if you exercise in a warm room when feeling relaxed. Warm yourself up by a little marching on the spot, with small arm circles, before you begin. If in doubt, first consult your doctor.

fibromyalgia

The National Women's Health Center estimates there are 4 to 8 million adults suffering from fibromyalgia in the United States, and 90 percent of these cases occure in women. Recent research published in the *British Medical Journal* found that graded low-impact (walking and cycling) aerobic exercise gave significant benefits lasting for up to 12 months in those who completed the program over three months. The Level 1 walking and cycling programs on page 70 should be suitable for most sufferers. Relaxation and stretching exercises have also been shown to have benefit.

1 neck release Good for relieving neck pain and releasing tension

Sit in a supportive office or kitchen chair and relax your shoulders as much as you can. Bring your head sideways down to the left, looking forward and without twisting your head. Now raise your left arm up and over your head and place the palm of your left hand on the right side of your head. Use medium pressure to bring your head a little lower down toward your left shoulder. Hold for a count of 10, then return to the starting position and repeat to the other side.

2 shoulder release Good for tense and stiff shoulders

Sit as for exercise 1 and lock your fingers together in front of you so your palms face downward. Now extend your arms out in front of you, still with fingers locked, and then upward until your arms are over your head (or as far as you can get). When you reach the farthest point that is comfortable, hold for a count of 10 to 20, then slowly return to the starting position.

3 shoulder rolling Good for tense and stiff shoulders

Sit as in exercises 1 and 2, with your shoulders down and as relaxed as possible (3a), palms in your lap. Keeping your neck and arms still, raise the shoulders straight up until they are near your ears (3b), then move them backward (3c) and finally down to the starting position. Do 10 slow rolls and then repeat, moving your shoulders back first (3d) before moving them up and then back to the starting position.

exercises for your joints

4 wrist flexibility Good for stiff, weak, or aching wrists

Sit or stand, keeping your elbows at your sides, and bend each arm so the forearms are out in front of you, palms down. Keeping the arms still, raise your hands from the wrist up as far as they will go (4a). Repeat 5 times, then, with the wrists flat, move your forearms around so your palms face upward, then smoothly move them back. Repeat 10 times. Lastly, hold your forearms so your palms face inward, fingers loosely bent, and bring your hands in toward your chest without moving your arms (4b), feeling the stretch across the back of each wrist. Repeat 10 times.

4a

4b

5

5 standing curl downs Good for relaxing and loosening the spine

Stand against a wall, with the backs of your heels about 3 inches from the wall and your back flat against the wall (or as flat as it will go, keeping a small hollow in the lower spine). Now tighten your abdominal muscles slightly and slowly curl your upper body down until all your spine is away from the wall, except the tailbone. Hang loosely for 10 seconds, then slowly curl back up again, using your stomach muscles to help you.

6 long back stretch
Good for stretching the muscles of the shoulders and back, and releasing the vertebrae of the spine and neck

Kneel on a mat on all fours and slowly slide your bottom back onto your heels, sliding your arms forward and keeping your head tucked in as you do so. When your arms are fully stretched and form a line with your spine, hold for a count of 10. (Work this up to 30 as you get used to the exercise.) Using the abdominal muscles, slowly come up from the position to a kneel with your arms in the air. Bring your arms down to your sides.

7 groin stretch
Good for tight pelvic and inner thigh area

Lie on a mat on your back (with your head supported by a cushion if you like), hands resting lightly on your chest. Bring your feet in toward your pelvis, soles facing each other so your bent legs drop down and out to either side. When they have dropped as far as they will, place each palm flat on your inner thigh near the knee and gently push the legs down a little lower, aiming to keep your spine from arching. When you feel a stretch along the inner thigh, hold for 10, then release.

exercises for your joints

8 lying lower-back stretch Good for freeing up a tight lower back

Lie on a mat on your back (with your head supported by a cushion if you like), your arms out to the sides. Now, with your head inclined to the left and the left arm flat on the floor throughout, lift your left leg, with knee bent, up and over to your right side so your left foot is level with your right knee and your left knee drops down toward the floor. Place your right palm on your left knee and gently exert pressure so the knee moves a little closer to the floor. Feel a stretch across your lower back and hold for a count of 10. Slowly return to the starting position and repeat to the other side.

9 hip flex Good for stretching out the large muscles that control hip movement and are often tight, which can cause knock-on pain throughout the lower body

Stand with your arms by your sides and your feet hip-width apart. Now bring your left leg forward and bend at the knee until your knee is over your ankle. As you do so, take your right leg back so you are in a lunge position, with the right heel slightly off the floor. Now press your pelvis down toward the floor (dropping your right knee slightly to achieve this) so you feel the stretch along the front of the right hip. Hold for a count of 10, then slowly return to the starting position and repeat to the other side.

10 long body stretch Good for releasing the muscles of the chest, shoulders, and abdomen, and relieving tension

Lie on your back on a mat, with your arms at your sides and your toes pointed to the wall. Now lift your arms up and back until the backs of your hands are touching the floor above your head (or as far as they will comfortably go). Shut your eyes, breathe deeply and slowly, and feel the stretch through the shoulders and abdomen. Hold the position for a count of 20 to 30. Move your arms out to the sides and slowly come up, rolling gently over to one side, then onto all fours.

10

1 bench press for upper body

Lie on your back, with your knees bent and your feet flat on floor. Don't arch your lower back—there should be only a small gap between spine and floor. Hold a dumbbell in each hand, with your arms bent slightly, hands at shoulder level, then raise weights vertically until your arms are straight above your shoulders as shown. Lower slowly to the starting position and repeat up to 10 times.

warm up and cool down

Before these exercises, warm up (page 74) and afterward do cool-down stretches on pages 75 and 82–3. If you have any health problems, first check with a doctor.

exercises for your bones Although osteoporosis doesn't usually make itself known until you are in your 60s or later, the process of bone demineralization can begin as early as in the 20s or 30s. It is believed osteopenia (early bone loss) is suffered by 16 percent Caucasin women in their 20s.

The most important alterable controlling factor in bone density is regular bone-loading (weight-bearing) exercise, which can be obtained some forms of aerobic exercise and by using either free weights or your own body weight to provide resistance.

aerobic exercise Skipping and on-the-spot jumping are two good simple bone-loaders for the lower body and can take only 2 to 3 minutes a day. If you suffer from arthritis or have been advised not to jar your joints (say, if you already have osteoporosis), then you can instead use a rebounder—a minitrampoline. Jogging, running, and walking (see page 70) are also lower-body bone-loaders, but cycling and swimming are not as your weight is borne by the cycle or the water. The only upper-body bone-loading aerobic exercise commonly available is rowing.

weighted exercise Research published in the *Journal of the American Medical Association* showed that strength training just twice a week cuts risk of bone fractures in older women. This appears to work because when the muscles contract during the resistance stage they pull against the bones, which in turn stimulates them to grow. Because most aerobic exercise is useful only for the bones in the legs, you should try to do weighted work to stimulate bone repair and renewal in your upper body.

The six examples that follow show bone-building exercises that rely either on free weights or your own body weight. The exercises cover the shoulders and arms, spine, hips, and legs, and you will need a pair of 1- to 2-pound dumbbells.. Do them every day, or at least 3 to 4 times a week.

2 press-ups for upper body and arms

Kneel on the floor on all fours with hands hip-width apart and feet crossed and raised off the floor, as shown. Keeping the abdominals strong, bend your elbows and slowly lower your upper body down toward the floor, touching the floor with your forehead. Slowly rise again and repeat 10 times.

2

3a

3

3 seated curls for wrists and forearms

Sit on the edge of a sturdy chair or bench with your legs apart, as shown. Rest your left elbow on your left knee and hold a dumbbell in your right hand with your right arm extended to the floor and the right elbow touching the inside of the right knee as shown (3). Now curl the right forearm up to bring the weight toward the left side of your chest as shown (3a), hold for a count of 2, then slowly return to the starting position. Repeat 10 times and then repeat to the other side.

exercises for your bones

4 | shoulder press | 5 | standing lateral raises

4 shoulder press
for shoulders and arms

Stand with feet hip-width apart
Hold the dumbbells with your arms
bent at each side of your shoulders,
palms facing downward. (4) Now
extend your arms upward above
your shoulders (4a), hold for a
count of 2, then slowly return to
the starting position and repeat
10 times.

5 standing lateral raises
for shoulders and upper back

Stand with feet hip-width apart and a
dumbbell in each hand by your sides,
palms facing inward. Now breathe in
and slowly raise the dumbbells out to
each side of your body, keeping your
arms straight, until the dumbbells are
slightly above shoulder height. Hold
for a count of 2, then slowly return to
starting position and repeat 10 times.

[6]

[6a]

6 plies with tricep extensions for thighs, hips, and upper arms

Stand with legs farther than hip-width apart, toes pointing out to 45 degrees and a dumbbell in each hand. Keeping abdominals strong throughout, raise elbows, palms toward floor, knuckles facing each other, so upper arms are parallel to floor and out to the sides as shown (6). Keeping feet flat on the floor and chest up, bend knees and lower body until thighs are parallel to floor (or as far as you can comfortably go). As you do so, bring arms out to sides and behind body as far as they will comfortably go (6a). Slowly raise yourself up again and return arms to raised starting position. Repeat 10 times.

are you at risk?

Some people are more prone to osteoporosis than others. Check the list and see if you may have a higher risk factor.

Female ● Postmenopausal ● Tall ● Body Mass Index under 19 ● Parent suffers from osteoporosis ● Caucasian or Asian ● Late onset of menstrual periods ● Early menopause ● Steroids, thyroid treatment, or some other medications.

If you think you have a high risk factor, you should talk to your health-care advisor about a dual x-ray absorptiometry (DXA) scan.

exercise for **relaxation**

What relaxes your mind tends also to relax your body, and vice versa—and exercise is one of the great ways of achieving both mental and physical destressing.

Just as it is hard to separate the relaxation of your mind and your body—the two almost always go together—when you exercise with relaxation as your goal, you will almost always find yourself reenergized and less tired, too.

This is because stress is one of the great energy-sappers, and if you replace it with calmness, the stress gap is usually soon filled with energy. So exercise for relaxation has much more benefit than you might at first imagine.

The foundation of true relaxation is the ability to breathe properly, a talent that few of us have, or even think about—and even fewer would ever consider to be "real" exercise. So, overleaf we look at this neglected function and find out just why it is important. The simple but vital breathing exercises will help you to breathe well throughout the day and during physical and mental work.

Once you have mastered good breathing, we can look at the typical "calming" disciplines, such as stretching and yoga, how they work, and judge what is best to do. A short guide to "quick" meditation will help you to clear and focus your mind.

And, although most of us imagine quiet, meditative exercise as the definitive "relaxing" exercise, even quite "active" work enables the body to unwind and calm down, so finally we discuss why you should get moving to help you relax.

The ideal relaxation program is one that combines all these three areas—breathing, quiet exercise, and active work. However, you don't need to spend a great deal of time on all of these, as proved by our 15 Minutes-a-day Unwind. Do it every day and you will quickly find you have programed both body and mind to relax almost to order, no matter what stresses each day brings.

breathe ...
The way that you breathe is a vital key to relaxation, because it both reflects and controls your body's mental and emotional state.

Few people are even aware of their breathing, or that they are not "doing it properly"—as, rather like the heart beating, it seems like something that should be completely involuntary and natural.

But not only is our breathing an almost instant reflection of what is happening in our lives, it can also, with practice, control emotions and physical reactions, and, thus, help to relax both mind and body. No wonder there are numerous sayings involving breath: "It took my breath away" (faced with an immense surprise); "I could hardly breathe" (dealing with fear or anxiety). How you feel and how you breathe … inextricably linked.

When you breathe in, air is drawn into the windpipe and then the lungs via two large tubes (the bronchi) and finally into the network of small airways in the lungs to reach the air sacs. Here the blood vessels absorb oxygen, which is the vital fuel for many body functions—most importantly, the brain and the heart—and which is carried around the body by the blood. Then carbon dioxide is released via the out breath, along with debris such as dust and other unwanted particles.

What is normal breathing? We usually take about twelve breaths per minute, but during physical exercise that can go up to twenty or more, which provides the body with much needed extra oxygen. Many people, however, have speeded-up breathing, which is shallow, and this is termed hyperventilation. The usual cause of this is emotional stress and/or muscular tension and/or poor posture and, eventually, long-term habit.

Hyperventilation means the body is not receiving as much oxygen as it should and this can lead to dizziness, faintness, disorientation, palpitations or racing heart, stomach pains, headache, muscular tension, fatigue, anxiety, and panic attacks. At times of high stress, the breath can literally be "held," for periods of time, without the person realizing he or she is doing this, which also causes a lack of oxygen to the brain.

In other words, improper breathing due to stress leads to a vicious circle of more stress and other negative symptoms, which can lead to yet more stress and even poorer breathing.

how do you breathe?
You might be surprised to note you are hyperventilating as you read this. Take a deeper breath IN and then OUT. You get the immediate feeling that you are releasing pent-up tension and your face relaxes a little.

posture exercises to help breathing

Practice standing with good posture Try this against a wall. Stand with your feet 2 inches apart, your knees slightly relaxed, your stomach and bottom tucked in, your ribcage free, your shoulders down and relaxed, your spine straight but with a light curve at the bottom, your head balanced well on your neck, without the chin pointing upward. Check that your pelvis is in "neutral"—if it tilts forward your stomach will tend to protrude. Stand like this and concentrate on holding good posture while breathing normally.

chest stretch Stand with good posture as described above. Now clasp your hands behind your back just above the tailbone and bring your arms out behind you as far as you can. Feel a stretch all across your chest. Hold for a count of 10 and return to the starting position. Repeat this several times a day.

check Lie down and relax with your right hand on your bellybutton and your left hand on your chest. If you see your right hand moving up and down as you breathe more than your left hand, then your breathing (at the moment at least!) is good. More chest movement indicates you have shallow breathing.

AT RISK People who have stressful jobs that involve a lot of deskwork or driving (both linked to poor posture) and long hours focusing on mental tasks (no focus on the body) are at highest risk of hyperventilation.

relearning breathing
Just as poor breathing brings a potentially long list of negative side effects, good breathing is an important exercise that can make you feel better, help calm you down, and help you to relax in both mind and body. With deeper, regular breathing you will be fully oxygenated with muscles that can relax. Opposite is a 5-step exercise plan for better breathing. Practice it every day to overcome your old bad habits.

5 steps to better breathing

In the morning and in the evening, stand or sit in an upright chair with your shoulders relaxed and back and chest as "free" as you can manage, hands resting lightly on the lower abdomen.

Do a "false yawn" to release jaw tension. Now breathe in through your nose to a count of 5, concentrating on getting the breath down into the stomach area. Breathe slowly out through your mouth to a count of 3 to 5. (The nose catches pollutants in the air on their way into your body, the mouth allows pollutants to be released from the body.) Do this for 1 minute, using a timer if possible.

2 Aim eventually to get your rate down to eight breaths a minute. Slower breathing is calming and indicates you are getting sufficient oxygen into your system.

3 Throughout the day, remember to do this type of breathing in difficult situations and when you feel tense.

4 Find yourself a key so you remember to keep checking your breathing all day long. The key can be someone or something that appears or happens frequently in your day. For example, it could be your partner or your work colleague, or the "new-message" symbol on your computer, or your cat, or every time you have a drink, or go to the bathroom. Every time this key happens, it is your reminder to check your breathing.

5 Work on your posture. The correct posture helps to release the chest muscles so the diaphragm can expand properly, and postural and stretching exercises help release tension in the head, neck, shoulders, back, and chest, which also restricts breathing. Do the long body stretch (page 103) daily, the exercises that follow overleaf and add on any of the upper body stretches on pages 75 and 82–3 if you have time. The suggestions featured in the box on posture opposite will also help.

chill ... Slow, gentle, yet deep exercise is a great way to help you relax in both mind and body.

exercises to relax

If you regularly practice stretching (such as in the exercises on pages 75 and 82–3) or do yoga (the positions of these exercises are based on yoga poses) or other disciplines, such as Alexander technique, Feldenkrais, or tai chi, you will soon find your body is less tense and you feel more calm and relaxed. Just a few minutes a day are enough to achieve this effect, but longer periods will also help provide other benefits—such as a more toned and supple body, and better whole-body posture. Back pain might also be relieved.

While you do the exercises, don't forget to breathe properly. When holding a stretch or a pose, breathe as described on page 111. Shutting your eyes can often help you focus on the exercise and relax.

1 wall drape

With a small cushion or towel under your lower back, lie on your back with your legs "up the wall," as shown, knees slightly "soft" and arms above the head on the floor. Relax into the position and breathe correctly for 1 minute. This pose helps you to release tension, feel less tired, and calm down.

Note: For a modified version, use a sturdy dining-type chair and place the lower legs, with knees bent and thighs vertical, fully on the seat of the chair as you lie on the floor.

2 the fish

Lie on your back on a mat, with your legs out straight and arms at your sides, with your upper back supported on a small cushion or folded towel, as shown. Allow your neck and head to stretch down to the floor. Relax into the position and breathe correctly for 30 seconds, building to 1 minute. This pose helps release your chest, helps shoulder flexibility, and calms the mind.

Note: For people with neck problems, bring the cushion or towel up higher to support the neck as well.

3 spinal twist

3

Sit cross-legged on the floor with a small cushion or folded towel under the base of your spine. Breathing correctly, place your right hand on the floor (palm down) near the base of the right side of your spine and turn your upper body and head to look over your right shoulder. Hold the position for 15 seconds, building to 30 seconds, breathing calmly. Slowly return to the starting position and repeat to the other side. This position eases muscle tension in the upper body and frees the chest.

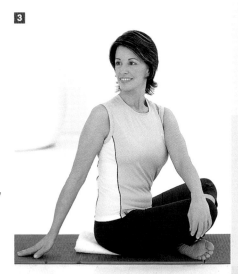

4 cobra

Lie on your stomach on a mat and place the upper body weight on the hands, as shown, looking straight ahead. Hold the position for 30 seconds, building to 1 minute, breathing slowly. This pose stretches the stomach and chest and strengthens the spine.

beginning meditation

Meditation can be a good way to relax mind and body, and is an ideal preparation for sleep, especially for people who suffer from insomnia or who have trouble getting off to sleep. There are many forms of meditation, a lot of which require more time and commitment than most of us can give. Here is a simple version.

1   In a warm room, without harsh lighting, and wearing loose, comfortable clothes, sit on a small cushion or folded towel on the floor, either cross-legged (which can be uncomfortable if you are not used to it), or with your back against a wall and your legs outstretched.

2   Close your eyes and breathe correctly into your stomach.

3   When you are ready, slowly say, "Aaaaah" as you breathe IN.

4   Breathing out slowly, say, "Huuuuummmmmm."

5   Repeat slowly for 2 minutes (approximately).

6   Focus on your body, starting with the head and moving down to the toes, aiming to relax each part of your body as you go, apart from your spine, which needs to stay strong.

7   Sit still and relaxed and try to clear your mind of all stressful incoming thoughts for several minutes, or as long as you need. This is not as easy as it sounds—every time an "outside" thought comes in, try to replace it by refocusing on your body and your breathing.

8   Open your eyes and slowly move up.

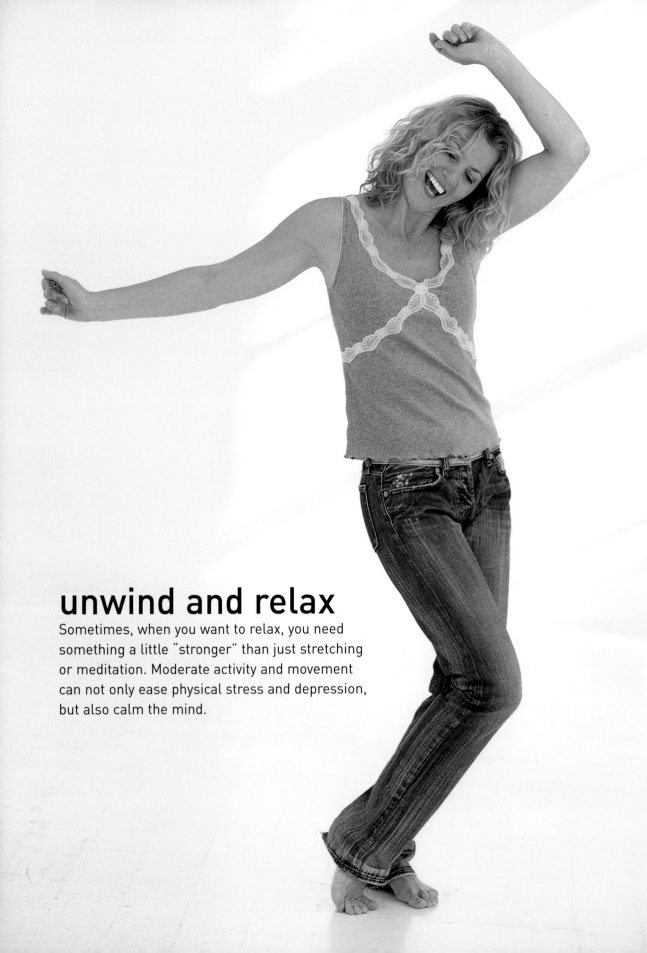

unwind and relax

Sometimes, when you want to relax, you need
something a little "stronger" than just stretching
or meditation. Moderate activity and movement
can not only ease physical stress and depression,
but also calm the mind.

Why does exercise help you relax?
The main reasons:

hormones at work

When you are physically active, your body releases chemicals known as endorphins. These have been termed "nature's painkillers" or "nature's tranquillizers," because they reduce stress and produce a general feeling of well-being. They can also ease depression and lift mood.

Intense exercise, such as hard aerobic work, can release anger and help to clear the mind, while more moderate but long-term exercise, such as a long ramble, can lift depression and improve mood. Research has shown that when people walk for 30 minutes their anxiety levels decrease by 25 percent. Whether you choose a 10-minute daily walk, 2 minutes' skipping, or a 3-hour fast cycle ride, you are helping yourself to feel better.

increased oxygen

While you do any form of aerobic exercise, your lungs are working harder to provide your heart with more oxygen, which is pumped around the body by the blood. This increase of blood and oxygen to the brain helps you to feel better, lifting the mood and, after the exercise, producing an increased sense of relaxation. Some activities that are not aerobic can also achieve increased flow of blood to the brain, such as certain forms of yoga.

dispersal of adrenaline

Adrenaline is the hormone released when we are under stress or pressure. It can build up within the body if not dispersed and, experts believe, is linked with an increased risk of heart failure and other stress-related conditions. Exercise helps to rid the body of excess adrenaline, which helps us relax.

mood manipulation

Certain types of exercise seem to be better for relaxation and mood than others. A crowded session at an aerobics class or an overheated gym might do less to help you relax than all of these:

● Gardening—good for calming the mind.

● Walking in beautiful or stimulating surroundings —good for lifting mood and awakening senses.

● Dancing—research shows music is as good as pills for lifting mood (disco-type) or calming (classical or ethnic).

● Sport—a noncompetitive sport you enjoy, such as skiing, rollerblading, or cycling, does more for your brain than exercise you find boring.

15 minutes-a-day unwind

Putting together all the ideas in the last 6 pages, here is a sample program of how you can use exercise to relax mind and body during a typical day:

8.00a.m.
● 1 minute's breathing exercises at open window.
● Chest stretch (page 75) for 1 minute.

8.30a.m.
● 2 minutes' skipping for brain and muscles.

11.00a.m.
● 1 minute's breathing exercises (page 111).
● 5 minutes' walk around your garden, or dance to music.

6.00p.m.
● 3 minutes' meditation.

10.00p.m.
● 2 minutes' poses 1–4 on pages 112-3. [Chill...]

looks for your
new life

We are all aware our moods affect the way we look—but the opposite is even more true. If you are looking good, you will feel confident and attractive; if you're having a "don't-look-at-me" day, you'll feel miserable.

And you can be attractive enough to boost your confidence at any age. In midlife, however, it is not enough just to spend time on yourself—you also need the knack of choosing products, styles, and colors that really suit you NOW. You need to avoid the "too-young" or "too-old" traps. You need the courage to let go of the "old you" and move forward, onward. And you need to keep up to date with the available choices, so all can be achieved.

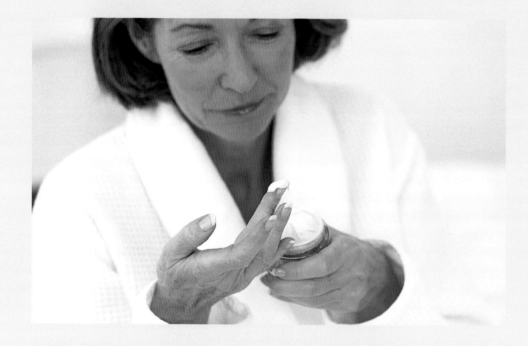

the way we look defines who we are

As we begin to age, however, we seem to take our outer self for granted.

In our 40s and 50s, it is so easy to look in the mirror each day, say, "This is me," and proceed to grab the same styles and colors from the wardrobe, put on the same makeup we've been wearing for years, and run a comb through the same old cut we've had since 1990. We have, we believe, more important things to think about today.

But, in truth, the way we look remains VERY important. As we begin to age, however, we seem to have fixed ideas on how our outer self should be—if, indeed, we have any ideas at all. Even if we watch our weight and work out to keep in shape, the "dressing" that coats the body rarely gets a second thought. And when it does, we seem to be led, lemminglike, toward the least suitable item on the fashion rack or the makeup counter. We then get it home, never wear or use it, and don't bother to try again for another year or two.

I believe we are so used to seeing ourselves that we can't imagine how, over the years, our essential self has changed. We see "me" in the mirror and, even if there is a small voice shouting loudly "you need a new look," we tend to ignore it. We have a set of habits—"our" skin routine, "our" makeup, "our" wardrobe, "our" colors. To change—for change IS, in almost all cases, needed as we age—we need, first, to realize long-term style solutions no longer work for us and, second, to overcome the natural instinct to hold onto the familiar.

We also need to gauge what is the fine line between looking "up to date" and looking "over the top" or—horror of horrors—having any connection with lambs, mutton, dressed as.... We need to achieve a style that is of the time, but still essentially "us." And we need to be unafraid to discard what is no longer right for our changing skin and hair texture and color, and move on. It is rarely best to stick with the same old hairdresser, who has "known" your hair for twenty years, the same clothes store, the same brand of makeup you have used since you were eighteen, and the same skin routine that kicked in at thirty.

New can be scary, but when your looks can make such a difference to your life, it is important to try. In Chapter Three, we help you to bring out the potential and possibilities in your looks—and help you avoid the pitfalls. For whoever didn't—on a particularly bad day—suddenly cry, "That's it! I'm going to have a facelift and I want it NOW"; or arrive home from a shopping trip with $500 worth of totally unsuitable clothes on a whim. Change and common sense are not necessarily incompatible!

First we look at the secrets of good skin—what makes skin good or bad? What works on your skin at 40, 50, or 60, and what can you realistically expect to achieve at these ages? How to take off ten years without botox, and how to look after your body as well as your face.

Next, makeup... you might need to throw out your old cosmetics to bring your face up to date and make the most of yourself. We give guidelines on trends, products, and colors for your age.

If you've ever considered cosmetic surgery, we provide the facts to help you decide, and discuss easier options that can be carried out in your lunch break. What treatments are really worth the money?

A good haircut can take ten years off you instantly—we show you how and also discuss coloring and condition. Lastly, we give you tips on repackaging yourself—the clothes shapes, colors, and textures that work in midlife for both men and women, and how to wear them. It's a fun ride—so there's no need to worry...

secrets of good skin

While we claim to love our wrinkles for the character they endow and the maturity they represent, it is estimated more than $100 per head are spent each year on skin products ... and many people claim to spend $75 a week, with the biggest spenders between the ages of 30 and 50. Here we look at what causes skin to age and give all the latest cures and treatments the once-over.

The number-one worry… According to research on facial appearance, the aging problem that most concerns women is wrinkles. No wonder the worldwide face cream market is worth more than $24 billion a year.

what causes wrinkles?
Genetics: your propensity to get wrinkles is to a certain degree mapped out by your parentage. This is the one thing you can't alter, however annoying it is your best friend never uses face creams and has a peachy complexion with hardly a wrinkle in sight.

sun exposure and pollution
Exposure to UVA and UVB rays harms the skin by increasing the production of free radicals (see antioxidants, page 19), which affect DNA, by damaging DNA directly. This damage affects the skin's under layers—the dermis and epidermis—and their ability to produce new collagen, which keeps the skin firm and plump (a lack of collagen means the skin collapses in on itself and causes wrinkles) and elastin, which keeps it supple. Atmospheric pollution also promotes production of free radicals and thus decreases the skin's self-repairing capability.

Repeated exposure to sun and adverse atmospheric conditions also increases dryness, and skin that lacks moisture is more prone to wrinkling. Some research indicates that if facial skin is 100 percent protected from the sun from birth, it can still be relatively unlined at the age of 80.

aging process
We all age and there is little we can do about that … however good your skin and however much you do everything "right" to keep it youthful, its youthful ability to repair itself and remain fresh, plump, radiant, and dewy will diminish over time. Around the menopause, hormonal changes often bring about a sudden seemingly rapid change in the quality of the skin.

There is not any cream or lifestyle choice you can make that will keep you looking 18 all through your life, so don't buy any product that promises miracles—but, that said, paying lots of attention to your skin can certainly help slow down its aging process considerably and help you to look ten to fifteen years younger.

using your face
If you were to spend your whole life not smiling, not frowning, and avoiding all facial expression, you would experience many fewer wrinkles on your forehead, around your eyes, and around your mouth. However, this isn't a desirable option for most of us, and wrinkles and lines brought about by using our faces are what are known as "laughter lines" and "character lines." They are, in essence, what make you you, and there is certainly plenty to be said for keeping them there and being proud of them. Although, of course, being cheerful and content might lead to attractive, upward looking lines, whereas being bad-tempered and miserable might lead to "down" lines—not so attractive. A point worth bearing in mind perhaps?

help at hand

If you're still using the same moisturizer or night cream that you did ten or twenty years ago—ditch it! Cosmetics companies have made huge strides in discovering what causes wrinkles and providing products to help minimize them. While some are hugely expensive, others are reasonably priced and might do as good a job.

Here are some of the wizard ingredients to look out for:

Antioxidants help to prevent free-radical damage. Vitamins C and E are two common antioxidants found in creams, while pycnogenol (pine bark extract) is said to be even stronger. Vitamin C also helps build collagen.

Amino acids These are the "building blocks" of protein, which is a major skin component and might stimulate skin renewal. The amino acid carnosine has been shown to plump up skin and diminish the appearance of wrinkles; arginine has been impregnated in jeans in Japan to improve the skin condition of wearers, while peptides—another buzzword ingredient—are an amino acid compound that stimulates collagen production, hydrates and firms, and helps to relax facial muscles, producing a "botox" effect. These peptides are patented, with names such as Matrixyl and B-neutrox.

Endorphins Hormones that might help relax the facial muscles and might also produce an effect similar to botox are beginning to appear in several new face creams as I write.

DNA repairers Various marine ingredients seem to help increase DNA repair and slow wrinkle formation—the cosmetic company Lancaster use photolase, an enzyme found in plankton. Another plankton enzyme is artemia, while other companies use salmon roe. Actual human DNA components, such as guanine and cytosine, are used in other, expensive creams.

Human epidermal growth factor (EGF) This is another form of protein, released when we are wounded, which helps to speed up the healing process by stimulating cell division.

Plant and yeast extracts Many plants are rich in antioxidants and other skin-repair boosters—green and white tea are now reasonably common cream ingredients, while walnut and apple extracts, Japanese pitera (a yeast extract), aloe vera, yucca, and sea algae are also favorites.

Retinol (vitamin A) This has been used for several years as a firming ingredient and often appears in cheaper creams.

Alphahydroxy acids (AHAs) These fruit acids might smooth out the appearance of fine lines—but avoid them if you have sensitive skin, as they work via a light peeling effect.

Many creams use not just one, but several of these ingredients, which might also help improve other skin problems (see overleaf). Choose a cream after reading the packaging carefully, and, if possible, buy a trial size or get a free sample.

and the other problems ...

Dryness Skin tends to become drier as we age, partly because the sebaceous glands below the skin, which produce oil, work less well. For those who used to have oily skin, this can be a blessing. Skin also dries out—in other words losing water rather than oil—because of wind, cold, sun, other climatic conditions, and heating, and these factors mean it is important to protect the skin with a moisturizer that both encourages oil retention and prevents dehydration.

A cheap moisturizer, containing a mixture of water and oils (such as glycerine, lanolin, paraffin, or seed or plant oils), will do the trick, but manufacturers add other ingredients (see above) that might also help wrinkles and other skin problems. EGF (see left), for example, is said to help maintain a "dewy, moist-looking" skin. Choosing a cream with an added sun protection factor might negate the need for a separate sun block.

Night creams are usually just moisturizer with a lower water content for a thicker product, and tend to have even more "active" ingredients added than a day moisturizer.

Sagging, thinning skin Sagging and thinning occur due to diminishing collagen and elastin levels (see page 121), so some of the creams designed to help wrinkles also help keep skin firm and plump. Creams containing proteins or amino acids typically offer firming and protection from sagging, while vitamin

for skin that looks 10 years younger without botox

- Eat plenty of plant foods, especially berries, apples, and fresh herbs.

- Eat plenty of oily fish, or take a daily omega-3 fish oil supplement.

- Drink at least 2 quarts water a day.

- Use a daily high-tech moisturizing cream and night cream (see the list of "miracle" ingredients opposite).

- Do 30 minutes' aerobic exercise every day.

- Get 7 to 8 hours' sleep a night.

- Avoid alcohol.

- Avoid smoking.

- Use a flash balm (at cosmetic counters) for an instant face-lift before a special occasion.

- Go two shades paler with your hair or have subtle highlights put into the hair that frames your face.

See also:
▶ going deeper, pages 136–41;
▶ lunchtime quick fixes, pages 142–3;
▶ skin creams, opposite.

what to expect at 40, 50, 60
... unless you work at it!

40s Previously oily skin can become drier. Pores on normal or dry skin might look larger due to hormone changes and slower speed of cell renewal. Fine lines are likely around the eyes, mouth, on the forehead, and between the brows. Thread veins might appear around the nose and on the cheeks as the skin begins to thin and the veins are nearer the skin's surface.

50s Skin continues to dry out and needs heavier-duty moisturizing. Wrinkles can appear between nose and mouth, and become more prominent around the lips and eyes. Jawline might be more blurred and a double chin might develop. You may lose fat from your face, making the cheeks look more hollow—a welcome effect for some, but not others. Skin is more sensitive and gentler products need to be used. Menopause causes loss of estrogen, which makes elasticity decline, sometimes quite rapidly.

60s Eyelids can become more heavily wrinkled and crepy, and bags might appear under the eyes (less common in people with good cheekbone structure). Skin is much thinner and paler than 20 years ago, and if exposed to sunlight tends to burn more easily rather than tanning. Use high-protection SPF and fake tan if you like to look golden.

Going on a diet to lose weight around this time can result in deeper facial wrinkles as the layers of fat under the skin disappear and the skin has lost its ability to bounce back.

C can boost collagen production. Sagging also occurs because the underlying muscles are weak and stretched. Dimethyl MEA from Roc and dimethylaminoethanol (DMAE) from NV Perricone claim to have almost instant firming effects by toning the muscles.

Loss of radiance and skin tone Dull skin is a typical sign of aging, due to cell renewal slowing down. Creams that cause a slight skin peel or dermabrasion, such as AHAs or alpha-hydroxy acids (AHAs—often described as exfoliants or clarifiers) will remove dead cells and make your skin look radiant, but they can be too harsh on older or sensitive skins. The US Food and Drug Administration is drafting guidelines for creams containing AHAs to carry a warning that they might increase risk of sun damage. My advice is not to buy these products—look in ingredients lists for AHAs by other names, such as lactic or glycolic acid and sugarcane extract.

Any thorough cleansing program with a gentle cleanser or soap will help remove dead cells, stimulate circulation to the skin, and make you look brighter and younger. EGF (see page 122) also makes the skin look more radiant by stimulating skin cell growth, while a light face massage with almond oil will achieve a similar effect. A weekly moisturizing face mask containing no AHAs will also help improve dull skin.

Thread veins – see Body skin, page 126.

Eye puffiness, bags, and dark circles The products most likely to help minimize eye bags and puffiness are special eye gels and masks, or eye contour creams and balms. Gels and masks kept in the refrigerator might reduce puffiness because they are cooling on the skin, and might contain plant extracts that could have a tightening effect. Creams and balms can help to even out fine lines, but do little to reduce bags and puffiness.

There is little evidence any cosmetic can remove dark circles under eyes. Dark circles always look worse if you are tired or stressed, and will also be worse after vigorous or prolonged exercise. They can also be an indication your cardiovascular system is not as healthy as it should be.

Spots, acne Although acne is often a teenage complaint, many midlifers suddenly find they have a recurrence, or get it for the first time in their lives. This is usually due to hormonal changes at menopause, ceasing to use the contraceptive pill, or sometimes to polycystic ovary syndrome. Although a healthy diet (see page 25) can help, you might need to use an over-the-counter cream containing benzoyl peroxide or see your doctor for an antibiotic cream or tablet prescription. You should also take care to cleanse your skin thoroughly (see opposite) and get plenty of exercise outdoors. Although sunlight has been shown to improve acne, you need to balance this knowledge with the damage that too much sun can do to your skin in other ways (see above). In time, most midlife acne caused by disturbed hormones should clear up of its own accord.

Lip problems As we age, lips tend to get thinner, flatter, and less firm, and small lines can appear radiating from the lips into the surrounding skin. This can cause lipstick to "bleed." There are various creams designed to help improve these problems and, indeed, creams designed to help plump out and firm the skin and ease wrinkles already discussed should also help lip condition. Lip balms and salves can help prevent dryness, chaps, and cracks. Several brands of lip primers are intended for use before applying lipstick, and work well to plump lips and prevent lipstick bleed. (See Wake up to Makeup, page 130.)

Flushing and ruddiness Hot flashes can produce blushing and redness, and the best solution to regular flashes is to spray your face with a cooling water mist from a canister such as Evian (a pocket size is available) and use a fan. A green-tinted foundation minimizes redness.

A ruddy complexion can be the result of a high alcohol intake or a healthy outdoor life, but some people are just genetically prone to ruddiness. Get your doctor to check you over, as ruddiness can have a medical cause.

Cleansing Even if you haven't worn makeup, do a thorough cleanse at night with a gentle cleanser and soft tissues or cotton-wool pads, or with cleanser-impregnated pads (using a separate eye makeup remover wipe if necessary) and then use a night cream or moisturizer. I don't recommend a facial toning liquid, even if you have open pores—it can irritate sensitive skin, and research shows, in fact, such products do nothing to help close open pores cold water doesn't do, and their effect is only temporary.

A once-a-week hydrating face mask is also a good idea for most people. With all cleansing products and masks, try not to pull or scrape the skin too much, especially around the eye area.

some more lifestyle tips...

1 Exposure to the sun is a major skin ager. If you keep your face out of the sun and/or use a SPF of at least 15 all the time, and wear sunglasses whenever you need to be out in summer, you should get many fewer and/or deeper wrinkles.
2 A diet rich in essential fatty acids (see pages 18–19) can help prevent skin dryness, as can drinking plenty of water.
3 Get enough—but not too much—sleep. Long hours in bed can make eyes puff up.

facial exercises

Do these exercises twice a day to see real results.

1 To reduce puffiness around the eyes: Use the ring finger of your right hand to do your right eye, left hand to do your left eye. Close your eyes and gently press a finger into the inner corner of your lower eyelid for a few seconds, then move a fraction of an inch across toward the outer eye, pressing gently again. Continue like this until you reach the outer corner. Repeat with the other eye.

2 To reduce a double chin/turkey neck: Sit with your shoulders relaxed and neck stretched out comfortably long. Now stick out your tongue as far as it will go, until you feel a strong pull across your lower jaw. If you look in a mirror you will see that the flesh under your chin has largely disappeared. This is because the muscles that support it are working to pull it in. Relax and repeat 10 times, trying to hold the tongue out each time for at least 10 seconds.

3 Sit with your face and jaw relaxed and look straight ahead. Tilt your head back a little and jut your lower jaw out slightly. Now smile as widely as you can—this will feel peculiar because it is hard to smile while your lower jaw is taut. Clench the back teeth as you do this. Lastly, move the lower jaw up and down slowly 10 times as you maintain the tilted smiling position.

male grooming
If your idea of vanity is splashing on a little cologne after your soap and water shave, maybe it's time to think again ... Time was when most men really considered it sissy to have any kind of grooming routine other than the very, very basics ... but if you still think that way, you're out of date.

Today the cosmetics counters are heaving with products aimed at men, and *Fortune* magazine estimates American males spend $9.5 billion a year looking good, and 51 minutes a day on grooming.

In midlife, in certain respects, men need to pay more attention to their "beauty" routine than women. Skin condition is paramount because, unlike women, most men don't—and probably never will—wear much in the way of the cosmetics that women rely so heavily upon to help to disguise flaws. Men also tend to have coarser skin and more skin problems than women, because of the different types of hormones that predominate in males. Shaving brings its own problems, including over-dry or sensitive skin, so know-how in that department is very important.

With care, suitable products, and just a few extra minutes a day, every man, at almost any age, can have terrific skin and the well-looked-after glow that only comes from attention to detail. And it doesn't need you to take out a second mortgage...

● Buy trial sizes of all new products, if available, so if you don't like it, you won't have wasted lots of money.

● If you are prone to open pores, pore strips (available at drug stores) are a good way to remove them quickly.

● Don't forget your daily antiperspirant/deodorant (used after, of course, your daily morning shower or bath). Although not too environmentally friendly, spray is better for men than a stick as the armpit hair prevents the stick reaching where it needs to be—your skin. It is true men do tend to perspire more than women do, and because of the underarm hair, they tend to get more potent body ordor.

● Don't neglect your fingernails—cut them regularly, bluntly across the top, leaving only a small amount of white (long nails on men are a turnoff).

● Avoid anything but the neatest goatee or perfectly and regularly trimmed beard. Avoid all beards—and even stubble—if your facial hair is gray, or going gray, as they will make you look much older.

● Shave off those sideburns!

● Regularly check you have no nose or ear hair (highly unattractive to women, even your wife), and remove it with a minishaver designed for the job. Also trim eyebrows—as men get older, their eyebrows tend to "bush." Pluck the brows to open out your upper eyelids, or get them done while you are at the hairdresser.

● If your brows and/or eyelashes are very pale or gray, consider getting them tinted at a salon. This doesn't take long, isn't painful, and the effect will last for weeks without anyone knowing your secret.

● Avoid excesses of alcohol and avoid smoking if you want good skin. Alcohol can give you a florid complexion with broken veins; smoking and alcohol are both drying.

● Younger midlife males can use tiny touches of makeup—clear mascara, for example, to thicken and lengthen lashes, or good-quality concealer (used sparingly) to hide undereye tiredness—for evening use only, though. A florid complexion can be damped with a green-tinted moisturizer.

● Don't forget to clean your teeth regularly with a tooth-whitening paste, and drink lots of water to help prevent stale breath. Floss daily and get three-monthly cleaning and descaling at the dentist.

● Check the section on hair for tips on hair care.

● Instead of using after-shave lotions to smell good (see opposite), choose an eau de toilette and splash it behind your neck/on your body/on your wrists.

shaving routine

1 cleanse Cleansing with a proper cleansing lotion before you shave not only cleans the skin but also helps prepare it for shaving. Shaving alone won't cleanse the skin properly, and many brands of soap have too high a pH level, which is acid and drying. If you tend toward oily skin/enlarged pores/blackheads, choose an oil-free cleanser; if you have dry skin, use a rich moisturizing cleanser. Either way, make sure it doesn't contain alcohol and use cleansing pads to apply.

2 shave Use a rich mousse or gel, not soap (see above). Some contain added moisturizers, which are good even for oily skin. Use a good-quality electric or disposable-blade razor (replace frequently).

3 refresh Splash your face with cold water and/or cleanse off last traces of mousse/gel with a cotton ball soaked in water. Don't use a toning lotion—these don't have any special pore-closing effect and can dry out the skin, especially if they contain alcohol. Shaving removes the top layer of skin (like a peel), which can cause redness and sensitivity, especially as you age, so treat your skin gently after a shave.

4 moisturize Smooth a good unperfumed moisturizing lotion all over face and neck. Choose a very light one if you have oily skin, a slightly richer one for dry skin— choose one that takes no more 30 seconds or so to be absorbed.

5 after shave? Don't use perfumed after-shave lotions! Many contain drying alcohol and additives that sting.

wake up to **makeup**

Makeup, well chosen and carefully applied, can take years off your looks and do a great deal for your confidence. Here we consider the latest advances in makeup and help you decide what is most suitable for you.

Why should I wear makeup? This is a question I have often been asked by women of 40-plus, many of whom think cosmetics are for the young, or who believe wearing makeup gives out the wrong signals.

And yet, if you choose the right products and colors, makeup can help you to look younger, look better, and feel more confident. Here are some of the advantages makeup can achieve for you:

it adds color
As we age, skin color and tone become paler. Discreetly applied, items like blusher, lipstick, and eyeshadow can return a young bloom to the face.

it adds definition
One of the first things you might notice about your face as you get older is that your features start to lose their definition. Makeup can restore this to thinning brows, brows with natural color that are fading, eyelashes that are more sparse than they used to be, and lips whose outline is becoming blurred, as the natural rosiness of young lips decreases.

it enhances good points
I have seen so many women of all ages who might be described as plain or non-descript, turn into ravishing beauties after they have put their "faces" on. If you have pale eyes, brows, and lashes, for example, even the most beautiful eyes can be hard to "see" when people look at your face. The right eye makeup makes them noticeable; a little lipstick can enhance a lovely lip line that normally is very pale and hard to notice, and so on.

it disguises bad points
If you bring up your good points with makeup this immediately takes attention away from any less good features ... But a little extra care with the cosmetics bag can do some additional disguising tricks, especially useful for evening time. For example, thin lips can be made slightly more full with a lip pencil and other new ideas (see page 134). Poor skin texture or uneven skin tone can be disguised with a good foundation; dark undereye circles can be hidden with concealer, and so on.

it can bring variety and fun into your life
Changing your look with makeup is very easy to achieve once you have the basics mastered. Using lipstick and eyeshadow (discreetly when it comes to eyes) to tone in with your outfit each day is an easy way to look coordinated and stylish.

it can keep your look up to date
As makeup is relatively inexpensive, it is easy to bring yourself up to date with the latest must-have lip/eye color or texture.

So don't be shy—let's look in your cosmetics bag and see what we can do ...

your cosmetics bag... let's give it a makeover! Here are three
simple steps to getting yourself products you'll actually use.

step 1—do a spring-clean

Take everything out of your makeup bag (and anywhere else cosmetics lurk) and sort them through. Throw out ANYTHING more than six months old that you can't wash. Makeup items such as eyeshadows and pencils, face powders, and lipsticks quickly attract a whole range of microbes that can give you infections. One estimate is that 50 percent of minor eye infections in women are caused by old eye makeup. Old makeup is also likely to be past its best in terms of ease of application. Foundation and nail polish thickens, lipsticks and pencils can dry out, and so on. And the colors/textures can be passé.

Wash and thoroughly dry brushes, powder puffs, and applicators that are worth keeping. Throw them away if they are worn, old, or not fit for the job.

Now throw out anything that is in a color or texture you don't like and you bought on a whim or in error. If you don't like makeup (even if it suits you), you won't feel good wearing it.

Lastly, throw out any foundation, concealer, or powder that makes you look overmadeup or caked. As you get older, less really is more, and you need a light touch with a cosmetic that covers your skin.

step 2—choose your basics

If you have anything left that fits the bill for any of the following six categories, then you don't need to replace that item. Otherwise, go to a good, well-stocked cosmetics counter and choose at least one of each of the following:

Avoid your old brands—it's time for a change—and spend time reading the labels ... cosmetics technology is improving all the time

Foundation The latest foundations give an even coverage without looking unnatural and many also contain conditioners, and antiaging ingredients, and protection against UVA rays. Look for brands and labels specifically aimed at women of a similar age and skin type to yourself, and which promise light coverage with a "light diffusing/light reflecting" effect (or similar words). Try several colors and brands out on the inside of your wrist. (If you have a tan, you might need to use the top of your hand instead, and buy two—for when the tan fades—rather than one.)

Go for a liquid base that doesn't sink into any wrinkles you might have; products with minimal pigment and a soft sheen rather than a heavy matt look, which can be aging. (Although some of the newer skin bases—by MAC, Guerlain, Clarins, and YSL—give a matt effect without caking or heaviness.)

Avoid heavy bases and very cheap products ... with foundation you usually get what you pay for. Foundation applied over a firming day moisturizer will look even better and will last well—you can even get light-reflecting moisturizers.

If you don't like, or need, a foundation that offers anything but minimal cover, go for a tinted moisturizer or a "skin illuminator." Avoid coating foundation with powder—use nothing but the lightest dusting of powder on the nose, if you must.

Eye pencil Choose a soft pencil in a shade that is no more than two shades darker than your hair, if fair or gray. If dark, choose a color that is up to two shades lighter than your hair. Choose a pencil that can be used for brows and for defining the eyes ... Kohl is too harsh for older eyes. When coloring brows, use a fine, feather touch with a lot of tiny lines to give a natural look.

Eyeshadow palette Choose a palette containing at least four colors and two double-ended applicators. If in doubt, go for more muted colors rather than

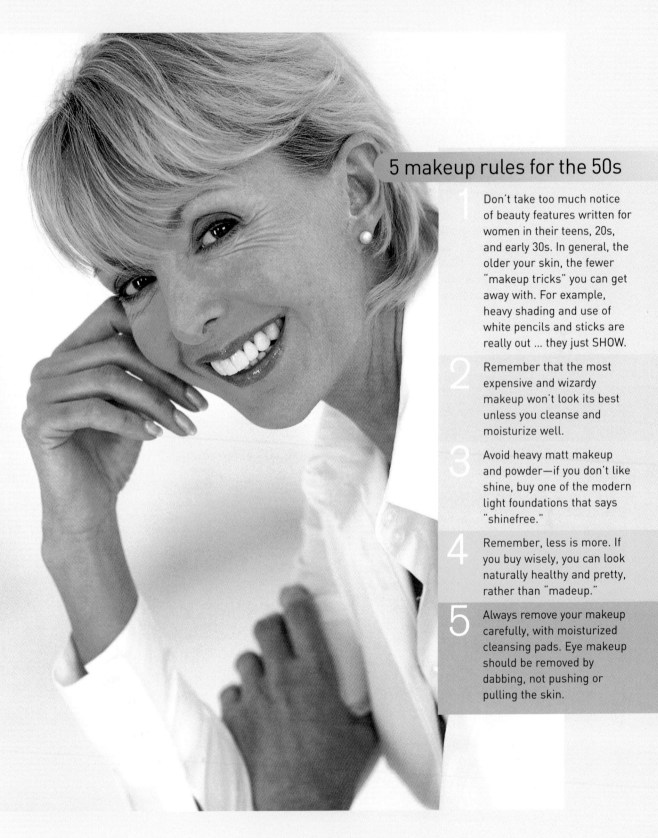

5 makeup rules for the 50s

1 Don't take too much notice of beauty features written for women in their teens, 20s, and early 30s. In general, the older your skin, the fewer "makeup tricks" you can get away with. For example, heavy shading and use of white pencils and sticks are really out … they just SHOW.

2 Remember that the most expensive and wizardy makeup won't look its best unless you cleanse and moisturize well.

3 Avoid heavy matt makeup and powder—if you don't like shine, buy one of the modern light foundations that says "shinefree."

4 Remember, less is more. If you buy wisely, you can look naturally healthy and pretty, rather than "madeup."

5 Always remove your makeup carefully, with moisturized cleansing pads. Eye makeup should be removed by dabbing, not pushing or pulling the skin.

bright ones. Avoid any shiny, frosted, or sparkly colors, which accentuate wrinkles. Cream (or, if you have good skin on the eyelids, pressed powder) shadows are best. Avoid anything too dark and blue if you have blue or blue/gray eyes, or green if you have green eyes. One color is usually enough at a time, but if you want to use two (on a large lid area), blend in very well and use colors adjacent on the color spectrum. Shades of peach, sand, cream, and olive complement many older skins.

Mascara Choose a lash-thickening mascara and avoid black. If dark- or olive-skinned, go for brown or dark-gray; if fair and with fair or gray hair, go for midbrown or midgray. Colored mascaras (such as blue or green) are usually a mistake for 40-pluses. Two thin coats are better than one thick one.

Blusher Choose a cream blusher in a shade from your color spectrum. For most women, peachy-brown and rose-pink colors are more flattering than red or blue-pink. Blusher should be applied, after foundation, with a light hand on the cheek-bones and "apple" of the cheek, and blended in well.

Lipstick Choose a middle-to-pale shade from your color spectrum. Dark lipsticks make lips look smaller —an effect you probably don't want, as lips become less full as we age. Straight red and blue-pinks can be too harsh for older skins and/or gray hair. Lippie with sheen is more flattering than matt, and make sure your lip shade tones in well with blusher and eye shades. OR choose a soft, blunt lip pencil (a shade at either end is ideal), fill in your complete lip with it and then cover with a thin sheen of gloss.

step 3—try out and add on

Add what you need for every occasion—ideally two eyeshadow palettes (never use both at the same time), three or four lipsticks, a lip gloss, a lip pencil in a neutral shade to outline lips before applying lipstick (MAKE SURE it doesn't show when finished).

makeup tricks

Check here for help with using makeup to best effect for you, and all the top ploys to get the most out of your cosmetics box.

getting clever with makeup

thin lips? Use a lip-plumping base/primer before applying lipstick, to add volume and help to fill in any cracks.

bleeding lipstick? Use a lip fixative/primer to help keep the lipstick in place, or use a lip pencil, rather than a waxy lipstick.

eye bags? Use a top-quality concealer such as YSL Touche Eclat UNDERNEATH the bags and use a very light foundation, one shade darker than your other foundation, on the bags themselves.

dull eyes? Go for glossy, acrylic-based mascara, such as Revlon Lash Lights.

tired eyes? Use peach eyeshadow and blusher.

small eyes? A lash curler will curl the lashes and make your eyes seem much bigger.

double chin? Dust bronzing powder under the chin area with a large soft brush.

dark circles under eyes? Mix concealer half and half with your light foundation and use this, then dust with a highlighter from a compact.

If you aren't sure of your color type, use sample sizes of makeup, the free testers at makeup counters and small pieces of colored material held up against your face to help decide what suits your best.

nailing it

Well-manicured nails on both hands and feet show you care, and they are pleasing and fun.

If you can afford an occasional professional manicure, so much the better—otherwise keep your cuticles in good order by using an old-fashioned orange stick around the nail bases after soaking the nails (in the bath or a bowl of warm water). Invest in a good pair of nail scissors that are really sharp, and cut the nails into a blunt wedge shape, rather than the old-fashioned pointy or rounded look.

One marvelous bonus of getting past the 30s is that the older you are, the harder—and easier to grow—your nails become. If they get very brittle, they can chip, though ... so nightly use of a nail-nourishing cream is a good idea. When I remember, I break a vitamin E capsule and rub the lovely oil into the base of my nails, which seems to help.

A French manicure kit will give you lovely white-tipped nails, which always look great and modern. Or go for color. I never thought I would say this, but you CAN wear blue and green on your nails and it can look brilliant ... but do bear in mind what you will be wearing as, if you aren't matching nail color to lips—as in the "olden days"—you need to match it to your clothes unless you are determinedly going for the funky or hippie look. If you are not brave enough for that, a colorless or flesh-colored polish can make nails look healthy and brilliant.

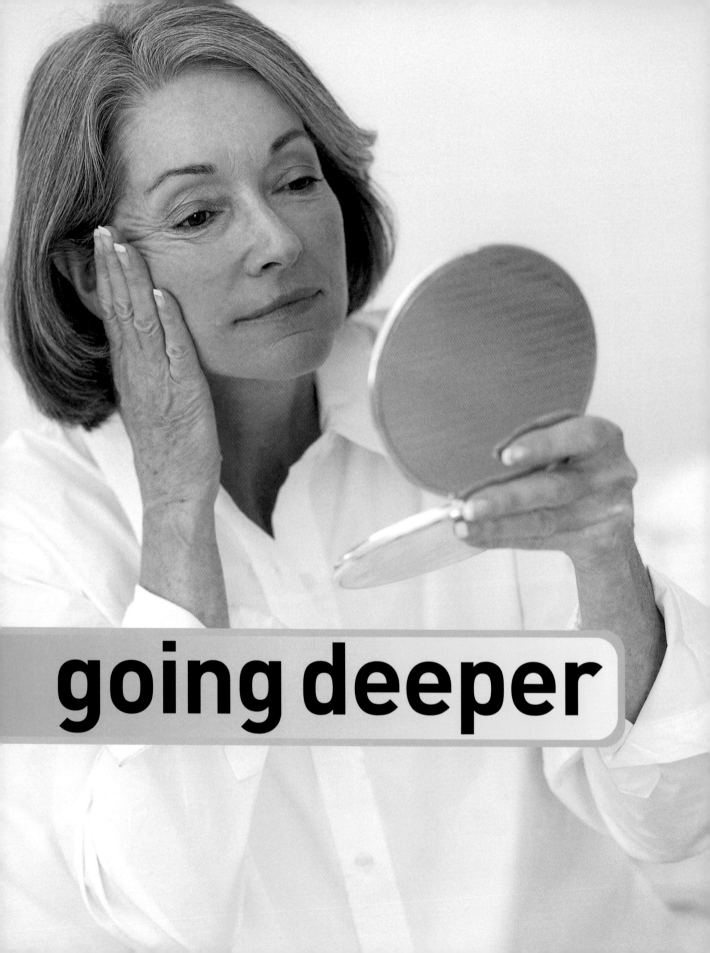

going deeper

Cosmetic surgery, such as facelifts and tummy-tucks, were once the preserve of rich film stars, but now most procedures are almost commonplace, while the range of nonsurgical procedures available to everyone is vast.

In 2002, the figure for all (legal) cosmetic procedures—including major surgery and smaller procedures like blemish removal—was 6.9 million cases.

Cosmetic treatment is no longer taboo—at least, not for women, although many men are shy about admitting to their facelift or chemical peel. Because cosmetic surgery is now so acceptable—even if not yet totally affordable—many of us wonder if this could be the solution to our own physical shortcomings. The cosmetic kings promise a magic cure for every single defect that plagues us from forty-something onward… eye bags, breast sags, jaw droops, stubborn fat deposits, spare skin, and so on, and so on. In other words, suddenly, the promise of youthful looks for ever doesn't seem far-fetched any more.

But even the lower-cost operations and treatments are still relatively expensive—many will eat up the cash that might buy you several vacations or a car, while even quickie salon treatment costs mount up if you sign up for a course of ten.

In this chapter we take an unbiased look at what these procedures entail, and whether or not they really are the magic bullet you hope they might be. First we give you the facts on the "big four" surgical treatments for people in midlife—liposuction, tummy-tucks, facelifts, and breast-lifts …. Which variations to choose? Will they work? What are the costs? Who is most suitable for treatment? How long will recovery take?

But before making a decision you need to know the truth about success rates and the dangers, pitfalls, and disappointments, so read the Top 20 Things You Should Know.

Lastly, I give you a guide to the popular lunchtime quick fixes—the nonsurgical treatments for face, skin, body, and shape that take only an hour or so…

the big four

If you are thinking of having cosmetic surgery, you are likely to be considering one of the "big four" ... the operations that most interest people over 40. Read our guide for all the necessary information.

liposuction

Liposuction (lipoplasty) is a technique where excess body fat is removed through a tube with a vacuum device. An innovation is the tumescent technique, which is similar, but the fat is pretreated with a saline solution under local anaesthetic, causing less bruising and swelling. Liposuction is primarily for subcutaneous fat (just below the skin) rather than deep body fat. Another new technique is ultrasound-assisted lipoplasty, which works more efficiently on larger volumes of fat and cellulite.

The best candidates for liposuction are people who are not greatly overweight, but have areas of the body where pockets of unwanted fat appears and is hard to shift via normal dieting and exercise, such as saddlebags and thigh fat.

Local or general anaesthetic is needed and the effect is permanent—fat can't reappear, because the actual fat cells have been removed. Full recovery takes from one to six months. The 2003 national average cost was $2,500.

tummy-tuck

Also known as abdominoplasty, the tummy-tuck removes sagging/loose skin from the stomach area and is particularly used for people who have been very overweight—in older age, the skin isn't elastic enough to return to normal via exercise. It is also used in women whose skin has stretched beyond the point of no return through pregnancy.

Excess fat and skin are removed and the muscles of the abdominal wall might be tightened. The effect is permanent—and performed on women only, when they have had their last child. It is rarely done on over-60s and not for people intending to lose a lot of weight (can be done afterward). Usually done under general anaesthetic. Average cost in 2003 was $4,400.

breast-lift

The breast-lift (mastopexy) raises and reshapes breasts sagging due to pregnancy, weight loss, or age, and is most commonly performed on women aged 35 to 50, preferably who have finished having children (additional pregnancies can produce more sagging even after the op). The procedure is carried out by removing excess skin and repositioning the remaining tissue and the nipples. It is often done under general anaesthetic and the results are usually semipermanent, but not as long-lasting in women with heavy breasts. Leaves noticeable scars, which a bra will cover. There might be permanent loss of feeling in the nipples. Breast implants might be added during the operation to improve overall bust shape. Cost is about $4,000, plus "extras."

facelifts

Basic facelifts (rhytidectomy)—where the skin was literally hoisted up the face and resewn into position—were the only option fifty years ago. Those having them were considered vain and ridiculous, and results were often not worth the pain and cost.

Nowadays, however, techniques have improved immensely and there is a choice of several types of facelift to suit most needs. The average cost is about $6,000, but, of course, depends on type. The panel opposite describes in more detail what happens when you have a full facelift, a brow-lift, or a SMAS-lift (lower face). All of these facelifts (plus other options that are available, such as liposuction to remove neck fat during the operation) are major operations, which will be painful and will need several weeks or months of recovery before the face is "back to normal," but the results should last for up to ten years. Other popular options are listed below.

Eyes Eyelid surgery (blepharoplasty) removes bags and/or surplus skin on the upper and/or lower lids and corrects drooping, but doesn't remove all wrinkles around the eyes—combined laser surgery can achieve this.
COSTS About $3,000 for full eye-lift, and extra for laser work.
SIDE EFFECT Discomfort, tightening, swelling, bruising, dryness, or tearing; sensitivity to light, temporary blurring or double vision.
RECOVERY Able to read after two or three days; back to work in seven to ten days; bruising and swelling gone in several weeks.
EFFECTS Permanent or virtually so.

Facial implants Implants can change the basic shape of the face, improving a weak chin, poor jawline, or cheekbone structure, for example. The effects are usually permanent as the implants don't degenerate over time. Cost about $2,000 to $4,000.

which facelift?

Traditional facelift: The original one where the skin only is pulled up the face over the muscle and fat, and repositioned. Most suitable for older people wanting younger-looking cheeks and neck. The one that is perhaps most easy to spot. About $6,000

SMAS-lift: This also repositions the facial fat and muscles for longer-term results, including neck improvement. It is especially good for wrinkle reduction, skin smoothing, and tightening up the jaw. It should achieve a natural-looking result. The skin, however, needs to have some elasticity remaining, so is most suitable for people in their 40s and 50s, or perhaps early 60s. About $8,000. The most popular version is extended SMAS, which has more effect around the nose and mouth and on vertical lines there.

Browlift: Lifts the muscles and skin of the forehead to eliminate sagging, minimizes browlines and furrows, and lifts the brows to improve the look of the eyes. Costs at least $3,000. Another type of upper facelift is the endoscopic facelift, which includes the cheeks, costing from $7,000.

Both these lifts are best for people who still have a good jaw- and neckline.

Lip enhancement Lips, which tend to thin out as we age, can be improved on a semipermanent basis (unlike collagen injections—see Lunchtime Quick Fixes, pages 142–3) by using fat (often your own body fat, which has less chance of allergic reaction), GoreTex (a manmade alternative to collagen), or Alloderm (see overleaf), or they can be reshaped to appear plumper with surgery. Both treatments need local anaesthetic, and prices start at about $400, but can go up to $1,500, depending what you choose.

Facial resurfacing Dermabrasion skims the top layers off the skin mechanically; laser treatment has a similar effect with a laser device; chemical peeling with phenol or other acid removes skin by chemical action. Each helps improve scars and wrinkles, and to even out pigment by encouraging new skin to form. Needs local anaesthetic and produces acute sun sensitivity; 2 weeks off work, and skin redness may persist for months. Prices vary from about $2,000, and more than one treatment might be necessary.

top 20 things you should know...

Before you go ahead with a cosmetic surgery operation, you need to know as much as possible about maximizing the chances of a successful op, and about the cons as well as the pros.

1 Successful surgery depends largely on the skill of the surgeon in question. Go to the American Society of Plastic Surgeons website (www.plasticsurgery.com) to find contact details for board-certified cosmetic surgeons in your state or region. Their helpful web site also provides unbiased pros and cons of various cosmetic operations. Your doctor should also be able to refer you to someone reputable in the field.

2 Try to find out how much experience your potential surgeon has in the field you are interested in and ask to see his resumé and "before and after" photos.

3 Check to ensure that the surgeon's certification is current and recognized by the American Board of Plastic Surgery (www.abpsurg.org).

4 Some doctors who specialize in fixing bad cosmetic surgery estimate that about 25 percent of their practise involves fixing the mistakes of other surgeons.

5 Remember that no surgery can achieve perfection and there is no guarantee that the results will look exactly as you imagined them.

6 Make sure you meet the surgeon who will be doing the operation and not just a "salesperson" or counsellor. Remember, counsellors are not qualified to talk to you about the medical aspects of your intended surgery, or whether it is right for you.

7 A high percentage of cosmetic surgery is done under local anaesthetic, where you will be given a sedative and then anaesthetic—via injection only—around the area to be operated on. If you are squeamish you might not like this. However, general anaesthetic, which renders you unconscious, carries more risks.

8 After cosmetic surgery, skin tends to continue aging as normal, so even though the effects of the operation itself might be permanent, you might, however, need another operation in the future.

9 Because the word "cosmetic" comes before the word "surgery," that doesn't mean your chosen operation isn't serious. Full facelifts, breast lifts, tummy tucks, some liposuction, for example, are all major operations, with the resultant risks and recovery time.

10 Commonplace side effects of surgery include numbness in and around the site of the operation, bruising, swelling, and pain.

11 The ideal age for a first facelift is between 45 and 55. At this age, you still heal fairly readily and if you leave it too late in life the results are usually not as good.

12 Permanent lip enhancement might be carried out using alloderm, made from skin from human corpses, which is washed, freeze-dried, and then reconstituted with saline solution before being implanted in the lips. Before having any form of implantation cosmetic surgery, make sure you know what materials are being used, and that you are happy with them.

13 Scarring from cosmetic operations is often played down, but, depending on your skin type and other factors, it can be permanently visible, and scars can be red, uneven, and raised. Poor healing and wider scars are common in smokers.

14 More people are going abroad and having cosmetic surgery while on vacation. South Africa is a popular cosmo-holiday destination. Prices are generally lower, but the standard is as good.

15 Complications of cosmetic surgery include infection, bleeding, blood clots, adverse reactions to anaesthesia, and prolonged tiredness. Individual types of operation carry their own risks: breast lift—permanent loss of feeling in the nipples; chemical skin peeling—skin allergies, cold sores; eyelid surgery—difficulty in closing eyes, blindness; facelift—nerve injury; and implants—hardening of tissue around the implant.

16 In Florida, a patient died after being injected with industrial-grade silicone that leaked into her bloodstream. The surgeon was charged with third-degree murder. This silicone is often used by unscrupulous doctors because it is cheaper than safer fillers such as Restylane or Nu-fill.

17 For men who have facelifts, there is a permanent need to shave behind the ears, where beard-growing skin has been repositioned.

18 After dermabrasion or chemical skin peeling, patients need to stay out of the sun for about six months.

19 Liposuction is potentially one of the worse operations for possible unwanted side effects. The risks include asymmetry (if saddlebags are done, for example, the result can be uneven to either side); rippling or skin bagginess where fat has been removed; toxic shock; infection and—with UAL (ultrasound version)—thermal burn injuries.

20 Cosmetic surgery might make you look better, but is unlikely to be the complete magic bullet for making your life better. And there is never a 100 percent guarantee that the job will turn out as you expected it to.

lunchtime quick fixes

Instead of using your lunch hour to go shopping or have something to eat with friends, you can go along to one of the many clinics or salons specializing in quick-fix cosmetic procedures that seem to offer many of the benefits of surgery without the time, pain, and cost involved. We look at some of the options from top to toe.

face fixes

wrinkles
You can be injected with various fillers to plump out facial wrinkles. The original collagen (a moisture-retaining protein obtained from animal cartilage) works well on lips and mouth, less well on brows, and lasts three to four months. About 3 percent of people are allergic to collagen.

Alternative fillers are restylane/perlane (hyaluronic acid), a thicker, synthetic gel and a less allergenic filler than collagen, good for crows' feet and nose-to-mouth lines; effects last six to twelve months. In some countries you can also get alloderm and silicone (not used so much these days because of side effects);. $200 to $400 for a session.

fine wrinkles
can also be softened with Intense Pulsed Light (IPL).

Botox is currently the trendy way to remove frown lines, crows' feet, and between-eye furrows. You are injected with botulinum toxin, a bacterium that paralyses the muscles that cause lines. Results are noticeable in three to ten days and the effect lasts three to six months; treatment costs about $375. New research indicates up to 44 percent of users suffer side effects, including drooping brows/eyelids, nausea, and headaches.

Electrical acupuncture (ERP) is claimed to treat wrinkles as well as open pores and broken veins, but the scientific research on its efficacy is minimal.

veins and marks
Veins on the face, blotchy skin and other marks can be treated with IPL—sometimes called photorejuvenation. Different wavelengths of light (unlike laser, which has only one wavelength) reach different layers of the skin and can treat thread veins without a great deal of soreness or long-lasting redness. Also good for acne scars, age spots, and sun damage—even tattoo removal. Several sessions usually needed; about $380.

IPL is now preferred to sclerotherapy as the treatment for thread veins (where they are injected with a saline solution), although the latter is less expensive and can also be carried out in short sessions at $200 a treatment.

skin conditioning treatments High-tech or new age "superfacials" (sometimes called natural facelifts) can make you look younger by improving the condition of the skin, relaxing or firming the muscles, refining pores, improving lymphatic drainage, and so on.

Treatments can consist of a facial massage by hand or machine with essential oils, cream that can contain ingredients such as aloe vera, seaweed, pitera, antioxidants, and/or masks (paraffin wax/plant extract/collagen creams), and/or treatment by hot stones, acupressure, ERP (see Fine wrinkles), electrotherapy, vacuum, steam, or brushes—to name a few. The choice is vast and costs range from about $50 to $150 a session.

Dull, rough, or aging skin, fine lines, and pigments can also be treated in the lunch hour with light peels, which remove the surface but aren't as invasive as deep laser or chemical peels. These light peels are often based on fruit acids or salt crystals, sometimes with pressurized oxygen therapy and a finishing moisture mask. It is sometimes claimed that these light peels also stimulate collagen production and can be called microdermabrasion. Prices are about $175 per session.

mouth:
Thin or wrinkled lips can be injected with fillers (see Wrinkles). The outline can be enhanced with semipermanent lip-liner treatment (about $600) or you can have a complete lip blush (filling in the line as well) for about $1,400. N-Lite laser treatment removes fine lines around the lips from $150 a session (several treatments needed).

teeth
can be whitened semipermanently in an hour, using a mixture of hydrogen peroxide or chlorine dioxide (bleach) plus intense light treatment. Costs $500 to $1,000, but not suitable if you have veneers or other synthetics in your mouth.

neck, cleavage, and bust

neck
Neck "lifts" are offered, based on similar principles to the salt crystal/oxygen treatment for the face (see Skin conditioning treatments). Cleavage treatment can also be included; from $100. A sagging neckline can be treated with electrical impulses to tone the muscles, but the effects are temporary unless treatments are regular. From about $60.

Botox (see Fine wrinkles) can be injected to remove wrinkles from the neck and cleavage temporarily, while collagen can be injected into the neck and cleavage for a slightly longer-lasting effect.

A sagging bust can, it is claimed, be lifted by a CACI contour treatment using electrical impulses to firm the pectoral muscles; about $40 for 30 minutes (10 sessions recommended).

body

stretchmarks
from pregnancy or having lost weight can be improved with laser treatment combined with electric microcurrent and ultrasound.

cellulite
There are several different types of salon treatment claiming to cure cellulite, but only endermologie—using handheld massage rollers and suction over a fine mesh suit, which you wear—has been shown actually to work. From about $60 for 35 minutes. Users also report good results with ionithermie (clay mask followed by electrical current) and pressurized oxygen treatment, although these haven't been scientifically evaluated to my knowledge.

inch loss
"Slimming" treatments generally rely on some form of body mask, which can contain one or more of a range of ingredients, such as vitamin C, coenzyme Q10, collagen, aloe vera, seaweed, algae, and caffeine, topped with a wrap of bandages or plastic wrap. There might also be manual or electrical massage to encourage lymphatic drainage via increased urine output, radio waves, or oxygen jet sprays. Experts say that no fat loss is possible through these treatments, only loss of fluid, which will return within a day or two of treatment. Useful for emergency treatment to fit in a tight dress, for example. About $40 to $75 for a treatment.

hands and legs

hands
Aging, rough hands can be treated with salt or fruit acid peels (see Skin conditioning treatments) or laser, which does cause the skin to turn red and form a scab, but is better for removing age spots.

Hot wax treatment can smooth and firm the skin, while oxygen booster treatment can plump up and firm the skin. For longer-lasting plumping, restylane (see Wrinkles) can be injected. Costs from $150 to $750.

legs
Thread veins on legs can easily be treated with sclerotherapy or with IPL (see Veins and marks).

hair today

Research indicates it is hair that makes the first impression, so it's no wonder that seven women out of ten worry more about their hair than anything else about themselves except their weight. In midlife things can start to go wrong ... here's how to have the best hair of your life. Clothes, makeup, hair—which do people notice first when they see someone?

If your hair looks good, you will feel terrific, because everyone knows the right style and color can literally transform you. A style can take ten years off your age, rebalance your face, hide faults, and accentuate your best features, as well as spelling out how you want others to see you—sophisticated, relaxed, or glamorous, for example. And a good color or colors can also take off years, make you look healthier and enhance your natural coloring.

Because of these obvious advantages of a good hairstyle and color, it is surprising that many of us, despite all those pounds spent on trying, don't make as much of our hair in midlife as we should. It could be that we get bogged down with the negative effects of aging on our hair.

It is also true as we age hair can need more love and attention than it did in youth. For some people, hair goes gray or loses its natural color, becoming nondescript. It might also coarsen, become more limp or start to thin. Some of these changes can be related to the menopause (or, in males, loss of testosterone), while in younger women hair problems tend to be worse in the premenstrual days. Good nutrition can improve hair condition, while stress and illness can have negative effects.

The good news, however, is that whatever your hair problem there is always a solution. Today we have a range of cleansing, conditioning, and styling products that will solve any problem, along with fantastic colorants, hardware that has come on in strides in the past ten years, and a wide choice of excellent, well-qualified hairdressers across the country. There's no need to settle for hair that is anything less than great in midlife, as the pages ahead prove.

fixing solutions What's your hair problem? Whatever it is—you'll find the answers on the next few pages.

As you get older, you tend to need different products and regimes for your hair. What worked a few years ago might not work for you now. Spend an hour or so in the drug store, reading all the labels, and choose products that most closely match your own hair problems (see Styling products, page 151). If necessary, have one set of products for "normal" days, and another for the times when your hair refuses to behave, such as just before a period.

You also need to make sure you have the best haircut you can get—even the best hair won't behave if you have a poor cut. Discuss your styling problems with the best hairdresser you can afford to visit and give his or her solutions a try.

"I want a style that makes me look younger"

The quickest way to younger looks is to go for a shorter cut—anything below shoulder level adds years to most faces, and anything below jaw level also doesn't work for many older women. If you really can't face cutting off longer hair, then consider putting it up most of the time—"up" hair takes years off you, too, but leave some fronds around the face, otherwise the look might be too severe. By the way, if you pull hair back off your face firmly it can give you an instant facelift by pulling back the skin!

Unless you have very fine or thin hair, it also helps if the style is "cut into"—creating tapering or uneven layers and thinning it out. Hair feathered around the neck and ears is also a good look.

Solid block styles all one length are aging, especially if your hair is heavy, when it "pulls your face down" by creating more volume at the bottom than the top. "Overset" hair spells granny if you're 40-plus (even when beehives and set hair are temporarily in fashion), so avoid any hairdresser who wants to give you anything that feels solid to the touch, is coated with spray, or doesn't have movement.

Choppy bangs are also a young look and can help to disguise wrinkles around the eyes and forehead. Avoid a center part, as this makes the face look longer and older. By the way, if you are dark, going two shades blonder or having highlights makes you look younger, too.

"I'm bored with my hairstyle"

Change your hairdresser. The stylist you have used for years will be taking you and your looks and hair for granted, and it can be hard for that person to see you afresh. Take along a few cuttings from magazines to show your new stylist some looks you like, and follow their advice.

To save too much of a shock, change in two stages. For example, from long to shorter on the first visit, then shorter still on the next. If you basically like your style, you might find that a change of color will be all you need (see Colorants, page 151).

"help – I'm going gray"

Although people generally don't like it when they see the first gray hairs, which seem to shout "You're getting old!", in fact gray—like blonde—can be very flattering for older skin tones.

If you don't like it, though, rather than try to deal with it yourself I recommend getting advice from a good colorist, as the best solution varies depending on the amount of gray, your skin, and so on.

If you decide to go with the gray, keep it well conditioned, as it can often appear dull. Some people also find, as they gray, their hair tends to thin out too (see "My hair is thin and limp," page 148). Experts say gray hair is rarely coarse, but most women find odd stray coarse gray hairs do appear. One or two can be pulled out (don't tell the trichologist!), but for generally coarse hair, a weekly deep conditioner and tongs or a straightener should help.

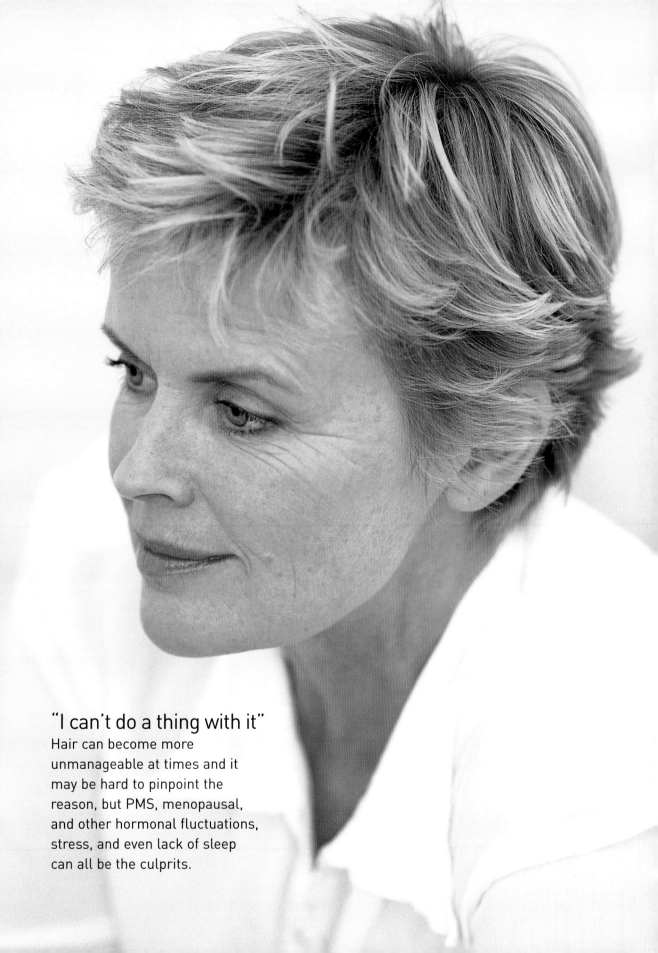

"I can't do a thing with it"

Hair can become more unmanageable at times and it may be hard to pinpoint the reason, but PMS, menopausal, and other hormonal fluctuations, stress, and even lack of sleep can all be the culprits.

"my hair is dry and frizzy"

Hair does tend to dry out as we age because the body's natural levels of oil production from the sebum glands reduces, which is why we also get drier skin. Coloring and bleaching can also make hair lose its shine. The answer is to change your products from those you may have been faithful to for years to those with more moisturizing and smoothing potential (see Styling products, page 151). Also use a weekly moisturising mask or hot-oil treatment.

Make sure you are drying your hair thoroughly when you style it. For frizzy hair, tongs and straighteners usually smooth the hair out better than a drier and brush, which tend to make it more flyaway. Use styling products, like blow-dry lotion, leave-in conditioner, mousse, or whichever suits you best.

"my hair is thin and limp"

Just when you want short hair, you find your hair is becoming thinner and more floppy. Graying hair is prone to looking thinner, as the white hairs that produce the gray are finer than your original hair. In fact, over time everybody's hair does thin, because the hair follicles shrink and therefore produce hairs with a smaller circumference. If you started out with fairly thin hair, the problem will be more obvious as you age. The actual number of hairs on your head will also reduce as you get older, contributing to the thinning effect. This is because the aging process tends to make the follicles lose flexibility and their ability to produce new hair literally dies. This effect is more pronounced in some people, partly due to genetics, but it might be staved off by good diet and regular exercise to increase blood supply to the scalp.

There is evidence that the contraceptive pill and HRT can cause hair-thinning, but not all brands do this. If you suspect this is the case, consider swapping to another brand. Thyroid problems can also cause hair to fall out, so get your doctor to do a thyroid test for you. Lastly, some antiinflammatory drugs can cause hair thinning if used regularly.

There are plenty of products that help give hair a thicker look, so swap to these. To help prevent flopping and limpness, use gel or wax especifically designed to retain your style (see Styling products, page 151). Also, use a lightweight conditioner concentrated on the ends rather than the roots. Heavier creams make the hair flop with the extra weight.

for men

Whatever your hair type, you can improve your looks considerably with some know-how and time.

the bald question

Although up to 10 percent of women have some degree of hair thinning in midlife, baldness is predominantly a male problem, affecting about 70 percent of men over 40 to some degree. In recent years, the "trendy" solution has been to simply give the hair a basic cut all over or even to shave it off completely. This can be a perfect solution, especially if you have a good head shape and the confidence to carry it off. But if that is not your ideal—what can you do?

In recent years, drug companies have developed treatments that are said to stimulate hair growth, but not everyone achieves good results with them. As they are not expensive, however, you can give them a try. Advanced Hair Studio's hair replacement system, for example, claims it is the nearest you can get to real hair without surgery. Lastly, there is transplant surgery, which is very expensive and time-consuming, but should last you a lifetime. Either way, it is believed that a real cure for baldness is on its way and could be with us within twenty years or so.

Whichever option you choose, please avoid the old-fashioned low-parting, combed-over look. Many men who have found the courage to abandon such a look—possibly even shaving their heads—have been amazed to find themselves looking decades younger.

styling

Just as for women, a good cut can make you look like a Pierce Brosnan doppelganger, while a bad one can add years on and/or make you invisible. Here are six tips to help you make the most of your hair:

1 Don't ignore your style. What worked twenty years ago is no good now. Fashions change (even in men's hair) and your hair texture and needs are unlikely to stay the same forever. You need an update if you haven't changed style in three years.

2 Avoid long hair (especially if it is thinning or balding) and, most of all, avoid long hair tied back in a ponytail—it is a real turn-off.

3 Avoid hair all one length. Even Hugh Grant has had a haircut, and doesn't he look better now? If it is thin, it will be flyaway and messy. Get it razor-cut and/or cut into shaggy layers you can mess up a little with some gel and look very subtly trendy.

4 If you need to look well groomed and formal, the cut just mentioned can also look that way if you blow-dry it with a small brush and use a little leave-in conditioner.

5 Make sure your hairdresser bears in mind your head and face shapes when choosing a new cut. Even small changes can make all the difference. For example, if you have a low forehead (not much space between brows and hair-line) and/or a large, long jaw, you need the hair taken off the brow and up to balance out your face shape; with a high forehead, shaggy bangs can look great.

6 Don't be afraid to use products to improve condition, shine, manageability, and the range of styles you can make within one cut (see Styling products, page 151).

149

hair help

Long gone are the days when the main help you could get for your hair was a can of hairspray and a noisy drier. So check out the goodies that are available—they can make all the difference to the way you look.

Whatever look you want, there are products and hardware to help you. Indeed, as you get older, hair often needs plenty of product to help it keep a style, although this can be less true if you start with a brilliant cut that suits your hair type. There are so many different brands—and within the brands different items—that it can be hard to know which to buy. So allow plenty of time to visit the largest drug store you can find and browse through the shelves, reading the blurb on the packs to find what most closely matches the effect you are trying to achieve (straightening, smoothing, glossing) and/or seems to offer the most help for your hair type (fine, flyaway, frizzy). But here are a few tips to help you.

styling products

Makers of styling products have lately developed an extraordinary range of names, but basically they can be grouped into just a few categories.

Leave-in conditioners, which you work in or spray in after you've finished washing and towel-drying your hair. They can be used after, or instead of, ordinary rinse-out conditioner, depending on how dry your hair is. There are leave-ins for all hair types, so choose carefully. They are particularly useful if you are going to use hot hardware on or near your hair, as they help prevent overdrying. If you tend toward greasy, limp hair, you might be better off avoiding these conditioners and choosing a blow-dry lotion instead.

Styling mousse or volumizer is good for adding control and volume to fine, flyaway, and limp hair without added "grease."

Styling gels, clays, and waxes are good for short styles with a modern look—tousled or spiky, for example. Combined with a decent cut, they can take years off you. For curly styles without frizz, there are serums you run through wet hair.

Glossers are usually poured into your palm and spread evenly through the hair once you have styled it, to add gloss and a healthy look. In my experience, these are best used on ends only in a small quantity.

Hairspray is still around, but better than it used to be. It can help you avoid that flyaway look without (if you pick carefully) being too "set."

shampoos, conditioners, and color savers

All-in-one shampoo/conditioners have fallen out of favor in recent years, but one or two brands are still available and are ideal if you really are in a hurry, such as showering at the gym.

Shampoos are best bought in trial sizes or sachets, if available, because what it says on the bottle can only give you a general idea of whether or not that particular brand will suit your hair. Price isn't always an indication of quality, either.

Conditioners often work best if teamed with a shampoo in the same brand range, and conditioning creams should be avoided if your hair is thin, limp, or greasy. For longer hair, condition the bottom half only. Sixty percent of us color our hair, and for us the new color-saving shampoos and conditioners might be a good idea.

colorants

If you've never colored your hair before, start out with a temporary color based on vegetable dye, then move to a semipermanent, which lasts about six weeks, and finally, when you're sure, a permanent. (Or stick with the semi for a color look that fades more naturally, rather than giving you a "grow-out" line.) Today you can even get a kit that you can use to give yourself highlights, so you don't need to visit the hairdresser if you hate that "solid" block of color that home-coloring always used to give. If you are trying to cover gray, you will need a permanent, and pick a brand produced especially for the purpose.

Home colors can rarely help you go more than two shades lighter than your natural color without bleach-type lightening, so if it is a blonde look you want, you are best off visiting a good colorist.

hardware

Even if it takes you a few tries to produce professional-looking results with equipment that seemed so easy at the hairdresser's, it is worth investing in some up-to-date hair hardware.

Older hair can become drier and more flyaway, in which case a combination of a light leave-in conditioner and straightening tongs (for a dead straight look) or a drier with a built-in smoothing brush (for a smooth look with a little more volume and curve to it) should work well. Straighteners have either metal plates or ceramic ones—professionals say ceramics are kinder on the hair and produce better results. Don't bother buying a straightener with a steam facility, which is unwieldy and prevents you getting the tongs close to your scalp. Straighten your hair instead when it is still slightly damp, for an even better result. Dull hair always looks much more glossy when you use a straightener, as it smooths down the hair cuticles and reflects more light.

If you have curly, longish hair, a diffuser drier used with serum is still one of the best options, as it removes the risk of frizz and flyaway. If you have wavy or straight hair you want to curl, get curling tongs with at least three different size attachments and—as the heat is direct on the hair and is held without moving for several seconds (unlike with a straightener, where the tongs keep moving over the hair)—it is very important to use a conditioning style aid before beginning to use the curling tongs.

repackage yourself

Clothes say who you are—or who you want to be. They can make people believe in you, take notice of you ... and have you believe in yourself. So don't fade away ... begin finding a wardrobe that suits your needs today. **Packaging sells.** Your packaging is the clothes you choose every day—and learning to "market" yourself by what you wear is a vital part of a new midlife image. You need to look great, whether the look for you today is tailored, casual, chic, glam, or country...

If you look good, it is easier to sell yourself to new people. First impressions count. Within a few seconds of meeting you, new contacts—such as prospective employers, potential lovers—will decide whether you fit in with their image of what they are looking for, will gauge your age, will probably even guess at your income, your social status, and your IQ. And a large percentage of these assumptions will be based on what you are wearing.

If you know that the clothes you wear—not only for special occasions, but also on an everyday basis—project the image of you YOU want to project, then you feel confident and you WILL do better in life. That image doesn't have to be "power," it can be gentle, feminine, masculine, relaxed, dynamic ...whatever you want it to be. And research shows that if you present your desirable image, even if you don't feel that way at first, you soon will. For example, you're feeling sad and lonely, but you go to an event wearing a "look-at-me" red dress and soon you're living the "carefree, center-of-attention" role you project.

In other words, clothes also help you sell yourself to YOU. They can help lift any negative emotions, while, if they make you look fat, dowdy, old-fashioned, tired, bedraggled, too young, too old, or uncomfortable, then they will make you feel worse. Look good —and suddenly you feel YES! I have possibilities; I still have a life.

Even if you are doing nothing more than spending a day at home, relaxing and reading the papers, your clothes can help you to feel good. Huge rewards can be had for a small outlay of time and cash. Worth doing? YES.

So WHAT to do? Repackaging yourself needn't take a great deal of time or even money, but you need to know what you want to achieve, so it does take thought and research. DO you need a total revamp? New ideas for home, work, evenings, vacations? What do you want to spend? You also need to know what dressing right for your age really means.

dressing for your shape—women

We all have features that we don't like, or imperfections in our shape. And however much you look after your body via diet and exercise, you can expect to see changes to your shape as you age. The tips here should help you to choose clothes that minimize the less good points and maximize the best.

tall and skinny?

Lucky you! You can wear almost anything and look elegant—which is why catwalk models are all ultratall and thin. Make the most of your looks by going with all the looks that plumper women can't wear—such as clingy cashmere, slightly cropped tops, boxy jackets, blousons, and thick tweeds for fall and winter, and flowing chiffons, florals, and ethnic looks for summer. Long skirts and flatties like Birkenstocks or ballet pumps look great all year around and, if you really don't like your swan neck, long scarves that break up the outline of what you are wearing do the trick. If you really do want to look shorter (why?), choose separates in differing shades, rather than an all-in-one look.

short?

Oh, the delight of being able to wear high heels without towering over anyone! But don't wear them TOO tall with skirts, or you will simply look ridiculous (with slacks that nearly touch the floor, they are fine). Shop at stores which cater especially for petite sizes so the fit of what you buy will be good. Go for fitted looks that will flatter rather than swamp you, and aim for a long line of color rather than breaking the look up. Shift dresses and coat and suit dresses rather than jacket and slacks, for example. Stick with small accessories—jewelry, belts, hats—and small prints or plains.

large bust?

There is no way you can ignore your bust by hiding it under voluminous tops so you really do need to "go with it." First you need to kit yourself out with some good-quality supporting and flattering bras that lift your bust off your waist and give you a cleavage, then you need to choose clothes that give a shape to your waist and hips, to create the hour-glass figure. To do this you might need to buy separates, as your bust might be a bigger size than your waist/hips and you DON'T want any top that is too tight. A V-neck is much better than a high neck. Avoid short jackets and go for well-tailored longer lengths, slightly fitted. If you have slim legs, go for shorter skirts and high heels.

no waist?

Best to go for the androgynous look, with well-tailored pant suits (there are many good brands with surreptitiously elasticated panels in the sides to allow for a couple extra inches) for more formal wear. Hipster jeans can be a surprisingly good idea, if they are not too tight, as they sit below the waist. Coupled with a blouson top or well-cut shirt, they can disguise a large waist very well. Any dress or tunic that skims the waist is good—avoid belted dresses and skirts, and particularly avoid gathers and pleats.

If you have a large waist, you've probably got slim thighs (the apple shape), so show them off in boot-cuts and shortish skirts (mini depending on age).

fat tummy?

Without saying the "corset" word, it is true that if you have a tum that sticks out or wobbles somewhat, while the rest of you is pretty OK, then—until you have the sit-ups licked—some supportive underwear is a fine substitute, available from any good department store (try before you buy). You don't have to be ultraconstricted these days to feel nicely helped around your middle.

Avoid clingy tops and any lines that finish on the stomach, for example a short boxy jacket or cardigan and avoid straight skirts or any skirts with a waistband that show. Also avoid anything tucked into the waistband, and instead go for skimming looks or blousons. Black or navy "absorb" a fat tummy and eye-catching detail around the bust and neckline also help

big hips or thighs? You need to

remember two things—first, balance your shape out by wearing tailored tops with strong shoulder lines or Ts, jumpers, and so on with wide necklines; second, take the eye away from the hips and the thighs by choosing muted colors for both your slacks and skirts, and brights, pastels, or patterns for the top, as well as big-statement jewelry or scarves, for example. If you have a good bust, a deep V or scoop neck can also be a good idea.

It also helps to avoid any jackets or tops that finish on the widest part of your hips or thighs, and go for slacks in thin material either straight-legged or slightly flared. Leather and suede will add inches to your hips—avoid them.

large? There are two main mistakes many

bigger women make when they choose clothes. One, they dress in what they feel is disguise, using baggy clothes and loose fits. This absolutely doesn't work—such clothes actually make you look fatter. Otherwise, they choose one size too small (or continue to wear their old, thinner wardrobe) in the hope that this will also act as a disguise. Straining zips and buttons and rolls of fat don't work, though.

The only way to dress if you are over-weight is in good-quality clothes. Sharp tailoring, which skims over fatter bits, can make you look 15 pounds slimmer. Dark colors can work well, but—with the right cut—so can lights and neutrals. Matt materials absorb weight; shiny materials accentuate them. Consider "plus" or "women" size designers.

Every woman has some best bits—for example, if you are plump you might have very young-looking skin and face … show them off with light colors around the face and a great haircut.

for men

short
go for fitted styles, single-breasted jackets and suits, pinstripes, suits all one color rather than pants with a differently colored top, shoes with a small heel.
avoid double breasted suits, turn-ups on pants.

narrow shoulders/ skinny arms
go for tailored jackets (made-to-measure will be a great investment), blouson-style leather jackets, generously tailored shirts.
avoid V-neck sweaters (in fact, most sweaters), skimpy T-shirts (especially coupled with baggy trousers), vest tops, raglan sleeves.

wide
go for dark, single-breasted jackets or suits teamed with similarly colored shirts and ties, or pale/bold shirts and ties, very good-quality tailoring that skims, not clings.
avoid jeans, combats, which can be narrow at the ankle and will make you look ever wider, double-breasted jackets and coats.

pot
go for pants cut with a slightly low waist and plenty of room around the waist and hips (tightly cut pants just accentuate your belly), hip-skimming jackets, roomy dark-colored sweaters.
avoid tight jeans and trousers, hipsters (belly sags over belt—horrible); clingy T-shirts, shirts that button too tight over the belly, double-breasted suits.

155

top 10 ways to avoid the timewarp trap

Nothing gives away your age quicker than a wardrobe that is years out of date or stuck in a particular era. Use these tips to get yourself up-to-date and younger-looking, without being MODAL (mutton obviously dressed as lamb).

1 Shop regularly—in other words, at least twice a year for main items of clothing and four times a year for small pieces. That way you're bound to stay up to date. If you're not near a good mall, don't forget the Internet and catalogues—or treat yourself to a weekend shopping trip with a friend.

2 Buy one or two fashion magazines a month for general ideas and direction. Don't just read the editorial, look at the adverts, too, which will give you ideas on which stores have the kind of clothes you would like and in which you would feel comfortable.

3 Enlist help if you are frightened of change. Whose look do you most admire among your friends or family? Ask them to shop with you or, if you can afford it, have a personal shopper (available at many department stores) to help and advise you. A freelance personal stylist might not be a huge extravagance once or twice in a lifetime. Try on things even if you think they won't suit you.

4 Always remember the clothes you loved ten years ago are highly unlikely ever to be lovely again. Lifestyles change, we change, fashions change, bodies change. Chuck out anything in your wardrobe that's more than three years old and which you haven't worn in that time—unless it is a true vintage piece, which can be cleaned and kept in a bag in storage, or sold. And chuck out anything older than five years, even if you have worn it in that time, except vintage ditto. Think of your wardrobe as a larder, with clothes each having their use-by date.

5 Look at photographs of yourself five and ten years ago. Is your style evolving, or do you look alarmingly similar now to how you did then?

6 Get in the habit of looking at what other people are wearing when you are on the train, in the office, in stores, or socializing. Become a fashion critic. What looks good, what doesn't—and why? Trinny and Susannah didn't go to college to learn about style—you can do it, too. Apply what you see to yourself.

7 And get in the habit of each day giving your outfit a critical once-over in a full-length mirror. Give yourself time to get dressed and to decide what looks good and what doesn't.

8 Twice a year, buy a few accessories—scarves, hats, gloves, jewelry—in the season's colors (or those of them that you like). These will immediately update your wardrobe of more basic colors.

9 If you wear glasses, update them every year or, at the least, two. Fashions in frame styles and colors alter frequently and, if you are still wearing frames from years ago, they will immediately date you. Choose an optician with a large range and devote at least half an hour to trying on as many as you can. Don't just go for something you like the look of—make sure they suit your face. Suitable frames can actually improve your looks. Tinted and/or reactolite lenses can also look cool.

10 Even if you can't afford to update major clothes every season, a new pair of shoes or boots in an up-to-the minute style will make the whole outfit look more now.

rethink your wardrobe
Once you've read the preceding pages you might have a clearer idea of how you need to revamp your wardrobe. Use the images on the following pages to give you ideas. Men, please turn to page 164.

"I want to look younger"
See Top 10 Ways to Avoid the Time Warp Trap opposite, which should help you to dress to suit yourself without looking too old or, even worse, too young.

Remember also both skin and hair coloring change over the years and, as you get older, paler and warmer colors, such as cream, beige, and apricot, might make you look younger than harder blacks, grays, or blues.

"I want casual, but tailored"
There will always be a place for blue jeans and T-shirts in our lives, but sometimes it is good to wear other types of casuals. Similarly, while you might be used to wearing a suit to work, you might just as easily wear something less formal without sacrificing a put-together appearance.

The key to "tailored casual" is choosing good-quality clothes that fit you very well, and think Gucci rather than JC Penny when accessorizing. The most relaxed of outfits can benefit from the addition of a well-cut jacket. Also remember ultracasual styles can appear tailored if they are made in a quality fabric, such as suede, tweed, silk, or linen. In general, avoid the tackier end of manmade fibers, going for at least a mix that contains 80 percent natural fiber.

"I want to wear funky clothes"
Well, it's partly in the definition. Are we talking Versace or Dolly Parton? Madonna or Pam Anderson? You also need confidence in your own sense of style. You need to buy and wear something because it is what you really want, and it says what you want to say about yourself. The chosen items should also fall happily into your lifestyle. Up to a point, you have to dress to suit what your life is, rather than what it was or what it might be in your memory or imagination. That said, there is rarely any harm in being bold at any age.

"I want to show flesh"
(see page 163) This isn't an age thing so much as a body thing. Daily workouts with weights and lucky skin might mean that at 40 or 50 you can show acres of flesh with pride. However, if not acres, most of us can at least show a tantalizing glimpse.

"I want to look sexy"
(see page 162) Sexy dressing means different things to different people. Some, for example, are attracted to under-stated sexiness—a complete cover-up with a hint of gorgeous figure underneath, perhaps—while others think sexy equals skin-tight, mini-skirted Lycra.

"I want to wear brights"
(see page 160) There's no need to put on the brown, or even the baby pink, just because you hit 50. Try on lots of stuff before you buy and begin with small splashes of color. Alternatively, if you've always worn brights and now wonder whether they are still OK, take your favorite colors (scarves are good for this), hold them up in daylight against your face and see if they flatter or make you look washed out.

"I want to look good on a budget"
(overleaf) Very easy today – thanks to outlet malls, chain stores, such as TJ Maxx, and regular sales at the major designer boutiques (Addresses, page 236). Even the least-expensive clothes can look great if you choose well and wash and dry them carefully. TIP: Cheaper clothes tend to be cut smaller.

"I want classic with a twist"
(see page 159) Classic styles can look very good, but if you spent years in the chain fashion stores before deciding you need to dress more like a 40 year old than a 20 year old, you might find the classic chain-store looks and/or the older designers boring—they might make you feel old. Seek out the classics that have their own edge—like Armani, Betty Jackson, and Dolce e Gabbana.

"I want to look good on a budget" As a general rule, if buying from the cheaper fashion chains, stick to basics and up grade the whole outfit with a few items with a more upscale tag. For example— budget-buy plain white T-shirts, buy last season's designer jeans from TJ Maxx, splash out on the best boots and/or a bag from Louis Vuitton.

"I want classic with a twist" If choosing plain classics, give them a twist with your own choice of boots, shoes, hats, scarves, and other accessories. Or wear half your classic suit with something else, such as the jacket with a chiffon skirt, or the classic slacks with a floral top.

159

"I want to wear brights"
Color can be good at any age, but it does have more to do with your own coloring and personality than with years alone. After a lifetime of black and neutrals, you might find you feel liberated and terrific in bright red or electric blue.

"I want to wear fashion"

It has never been easier to look fashionable at any age. The line you need to draw is between fashion that suits you and fashion you are wearing for any other reason—for example, because you saw a celeb wearing it or the magazines decree it is the latest length, shape, and so on. Although some women in their 40s and 50s can get away with high fashion of any kind, most need to go down a more classic route, adding elements of current trends, or else choose calmed-down versions of the wilder hot looks.

"I want to look sexy"
If you're aiming to do "sexy," you need to be sure of why you're doing it, to feel totally happy in your chosen outfit and to be sure the message you're giving out is the right one for you. If you don't want "skin-tight mini" sexy, dress up daytime clothes for the evening with more glam accessories and shoes.

"I want to show flesh"

There's no reason why you can't wear a miniskirt in the summer, or split skirt in the evening, if you have fabulous legs (which, it is always said patronizingly, are the "last things to go" as we age!). Cleavage can also be great. And take a look at your back in the mirror—it might well be worth showing off.

The best rule is that for every bit of flesh you show, cover something else up. For example, cleavage on display equals long skirt and/or long sleeves; miniskirt equals polo neck.

163

and for men If your idea of taking a fashion risk is buying a sweatshirt in the sales, take time to bring new life into your wardrobe.

It is said that many men aged over 45 never set foot inside a male boutique or store, feeling fashion is for females and someone else will shop for them if there is an emergency (weight gain renders complete wardrobe useless; everything has fallen to pieces in the wash; wedding or job interview to attend).

And yet … if a man does have a proper makeover, he always ends up with a bashful grin of real delight. "I DO look good!" "I CAN still play the game!" Just one day of your life is all it might take to achieve near miracles, so if you want to give it a try, here's a six-point plan:

1 Go through your existing wardrobe (I won't use the word "current" as it probably isn't) and be ruthless, trying things on if necessary. Put into a garbage bag everything that is old, tired-looking, out of shape, bedraggled, worn, stained, shrunk, discolored. In the bag also goes anything that is unflattering (try on!) for you in shape (see page 155), color, material, or in any other way. Ditto everything that is too tight, too small, too short—the only possible exception is if you are currently losing weight.

If there is anything left, sort it through and chuck out what is dated—although men's fashion moves slowly, over five years old and it needs chucking (classically tailored top-quality suits and jackets excepted). Anyway, you need a change, don't you?

Lastly, discard anything that is too teenage or too dotage for you. Put it on. Do you look like you're trying to be your son? Or your father? If not sure, ask your partner. Take the bags immediately to the dump so you aren't tempted to put everything back.

2 List your purchase priorities according to your lifestyle (Mostly casual? Work? Sporting? Home wear? Travel?) and what is left in your wardrobe.

This could be a new suit, two or three shirts, three ties, two heavyweight sweaters, two lightweight cotton sweaters, two pairs of tailored casual pants, one pair jeans, three T-shirts, two pairs shoes, and two belts.

Bear in mind the current season and, if you can't afford to buy a lot, buy half this season and half the next. This will also help you keep up to date.

3 Take your measurements (with help): neck, chest, waist, hips, inner leg. Write them down.

4 Decide where, when, and how to shop. Nothing beats trying things on, so real stores are preferable to mail order or Internet (although, of course, you can return unsuitable items and these methods can be good for some people). Department stores are usually good on range of prices, labels, and styles, and if you are an uncomfortable or virgin shopper, smaller boutiques and stores can be daunting. Some larger stores offer the assistance of a personal shopper, which can be free or you may pay a fee (usually well worth it). Or, take an acquaintance with a good sense of style who knows you well.

5 Armed with your shopping list and your size list, shop. Set aside a minimum of several hours to do your shopping and try hard to make sure your chosen pieces coordinate with each other, so you will look put together and you can mix and match.

6 Begin wearing your new clothes straight away—they aren't to be saved for a rainy day. And remember now to shop AT LEAST once a year. It's only fashion … but you know you like it really.

work or formal wear

You might be amazed at the range of suits now available—colors, materials, and styles to suit everyone. But it could be time to splash out on a made-to-measure or couture suit—go on, spoil yourself. If you travel abroad $750 might be enough; otherwise budget up to $2,000. Go tieless for midformal, and use shoes to make your outfit more or less formal as the occasion demands.

jeans for men

Many times I have heard it said that people over 50 (sometimes even 40) shouldn't wear jeans—and yet they are a mainstay of nearly everyone's wardrobe, whatever your age, male or female. Men, in particular, would be lost without their denims ... So if you've ever had anyone sneer a little at your post-40 body in your Levi's, here are some tips to bear in mind:

● Buy a new pair of blue jeans at least once a year—only pre-25s can get away with rips and fraying, without looking like a homeless person.

● Pay attention to cut. If you have a large belly, choose jeans with a slight flare. Avoid hipsters unless you have a perfect figure. Don't buy them too tight on the leg unless you have a perfect figure, with long, lean legs.

● Dark denim looks better as you get older.

● Try something new—jeans in black denim are attractive and, teamed with a good jacket or well-cut shirt, can take you almost anywhere.

● All jeans look much more attractive if worn with a good-quality leather belt.

● Don't wear trainers with your jeans all the time ... loafers can look terrific and expensive leather can improve any color of jeans.

● Avoid white socks. Wear either no socks (summer) or socks to match your jeans or shoes.

casual When going for your casual look(s), think about your coloring. Gray hair suits light and dark gray, navy, taupe, olive, stone, blue tints, and ice colors. Reddish skin tones can be dampened with cream, beige, camel, and taupe. Try polos rather than T-shirts some of the time, and go for the new breed of casual shoes that mix the comfort and practicality of trainers with tailored looks.

well-being
for your
newlife

With few exceptions, life is as good as YOU feel … research shows good health can improve not only your physical and mental capabilities, but also your appearance and your outlook. So if you want to enjoy yourself, not only in the present, but also for the rest of your days, it is vital to look after yourself.

True good health comes from a holistic approach, and in this section we look at all the aspects of well-being that particularly affect people in midlife. From the female menopause and male andropause, and the sexual dilemmas many people face at this time, through to problems such as tiredness, depression, and stress, and onto the life-threatening diseases like cancer and diabetes, in Chapter 4 you will find the inspiration—and the answers – to help you make midlife your healthiest time yet.

if you take some care now, you can live not only a longer life, but also one that gives you more independence, enjoyment, contentment, excitement, and so on.

While a hundred years ago you were likely to end your life at around the age of 50, in the twenty-first century midlifers can expect to live on for at least another thirty years, with unprecedented numbers of men and women now also reaching their 90s and the magic 100-plus.

Even better news is that, according to American research, the period of "old age" (with ill health and disability) is becoming shorter and shorter, so our "middle age" now extends to at least the age of 70.

In other words—despite all the doom and gloom and health scares—you can probably look forward to a long and healthy life ahead of you even if you are already into your 50s or 60s. To maximize this potential, HOWEVER, you do need to look after yourself.

Chapter 4 is all about making the most of what you have, healthwise, and minimizing the problems. For women the major physical "event" of midlife is the menopause. We look at what actually happens and the pros and cons of HRT and alternative treatments. And it is not just women who are affected by physical changes in midlife.

At this time, it is common for the libido to diminish, and a poor sex life can spoil the best of relationships. The second section in the chapter answers questions, such as, "What is normal?" "What can be done to overcome libido problems in both men and women?" Poor libido can often be caused by the health problems that are common in midlife, and in the pages that follow we examine these. One of the major cries I hear is "I am tired/exhausted/ have no energy." Although a frequent problem, lack of energy and sparkle is not insurmountable, so we look at solutions, including how to get a good night's sleep.

Body aches and pains can be a depressing and debilitating arrival in midlife. We examine how to manage—or even largely avoid—arthritis and other muscular/skeletal problems, and look at what—apart from diet and exercise (already discussed)—can be done to protect your bones against osteoporosis.

Many people over 45 or so tell me they can no longer take for granted their digestive system will operate smoothly and without complaint. Irritable bowel, ulcers, and heartburn are three "spoilers" that can all be contained, as you will see. If you want to live a long and healthy life, you need to minimize your risk of getting one of the "big three" diseases of middle age—heart disease, cancer, and diabetes. You also need to consider your intake of alcohol, possibly tackle a nicotine habit, and even get to grips with your intake of drugs—whether they are over-the-counter, prescribed, or illegal! Giving up a habit is easier than you might think...

Lastly, you can find help for your state of mind. Anxiety, depression, stress, and poor memory are all common in midlife, but they can be tackled and controlled. Well-being is what you can have, and what you need, if you are to also enjoy the great benefits of those later midlife years ... time, freedom, and independence.

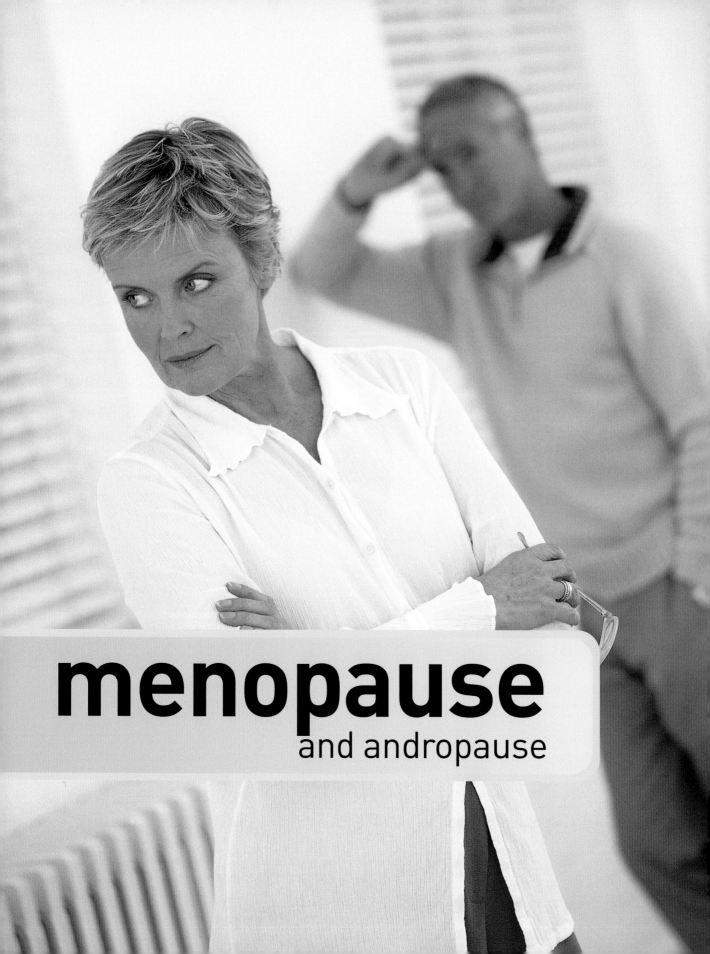

menopause
and andropause

In their late 40s or early 50s, most women (and many men) go through far-reaching changes, both physical and emotional. If you understand and manage what is happening to you, the menopausal/andropausal years—and those that follow—can be a change for the better.

Most women begin perimenopause in their late 40s, with periods becoming erratic, which leads—on average by the age of 51—to menopause itself, when periods and reproductive life cease.

The male menopause is a much-debated topic, with many professionals believing it doesn't exist, but very many men are very convinced it certainly does. Men might not have periods to lose, but they can testify that night sweats, hot flashes, lack of libido, and other annoying symptoms most definitely do happen.

We look at the side effects of both male and female menopause and see how best you can cope during this time which, let's face it, is a big chunk out of your life. If you ask doctors how long your symptoms, like hot flashes, will last, most will say three to four years. In truth, however, they can last for much longer than that, and often do.

We also discuss the long-term effects that going through the "change," as it is sometimes called, can bring. There is much research indicating that after menopause women are more susceptible to illnesses, such as heart disease and breast cancer. Many women put on a lot of weight in these years, although some scientists still believe there is no hormonal link causing this to happen. Most people are also aware that, when periods cease, bone loss accelerates and this can lead to the debilitating disease osteoporosis.

Over the past thirty years or more, hormone replacement therapy (HRT) has been heralded as the complete answer to beating menopausal symptoms in women, and lowering the long-term health risks. In recent years, however, there has been a move away from HRT, after fears it can cause its own health problems. We look at the facts, and also at the many alternative natural and herbal remedies available. They can be natural—but do they work? While for men, are there ANY remedies they can buy for their own andropausal symptoms?

In all this uncertainty and confusion, what is certain is that most people find ways to survive, with their sanity intact, and agree life is as good as ever, during the menopausal years and after.

facts about menopause
Many of us have little or no conception of what happens before and during menopause. Here we look at what it really means.

women

The phase leading up to the female menopause, which often begins in the late 40s and lasts between two and five years in most cases, is called perimenopause. During this time a woman's periods become more erratic and gaps betweenthem become longer. Many women begin to have symptoms such as headaches or feelings of irritability or low mood. The "midlife crisis" is on its way!

As perimenopause nears the actual menopause, other symptoms like hot flashes, night sweats, and joint aches and pains can arrive. Levels of the hormones estrogen and progesterone fall to about 80 percent of what they were before perimenopause began, as egg production ceases and the ovaries become redundant. Finally, menopause is officially defined as 12 months from the date of your last period, after which naturally occurring pregnancy is no longer possible.

The average age for menopause is 51, although it can happen much earlier—before 45 it is described as premature menopause.

men

The existence of the male menopause (andropause) is a subject of international debate. The pro-andropause theorists claim that about the age of 50 up to 50 percent of men experience a noticeable or sharp decline in androgen levels (the male sex hormones, which include testosterone), rather than a gentle decline throughout mid- and later life, which is the pattern that many endocrinologists perceive in most males.

Symptoms such as decreased sex drive (see pages 178–83), low sperm count, fatigue, night sweats, decline in drive and ambition, and depression have been reported, while the antiandropause lobby say these symptoms are probably psychological and/or caused by unhealthy living in middle age.

However, even the "anti" lobby agrees that about 5 percent of midlife males do suffer a severe dip in hormonal levels over a short period of time, which can result in loss of libido, muscle, and hair, as well as diminished bone density—leaving some men as prone to osteoporosis as postmenopausal women.

Whether or not a medical andropause is true for most men—and the issue is far from decided—there is no doubt many do experience a midlife physical and emotional crisis.

long-term consequences

While the more debilitating symptoms of female menopause (described in the panel opposite) are immediately obvious and easy to quantify, in the long-term as well, menopause can have far-reaching effects on health.

While premenopausal women have natural protection (via estrogen) from heart disease, once estrogen levels drop after menopause, they are as at risk of heart and circulatory problems as men.

Breast cancer and other cancers also increase significantly in postmenopausal women, while the accelerated bone loss causes a vastly increased risk of developing steoporosis in later midlife and old age. Many women gain a significant amount of weight during menopause and in the few years afterward and, again, medical opinion is divided over whether this is directly related to the hormonal changes—which could slow down the metabolic rate—or is just a lifestyle factor about this age.

Sexual function can be affected, because the loss of estrogen means the vaginal wall becomes thinner, less elastic, and less moist, while sexual appetite can also be diminished—for additional discussion on these problems, see pages 178–83.

symptoms of menopause

A woman going through perimenopause or menopause can experience some or all of these symptoms—or, occasionally, none at all—which can be sporadic and varying in intensity. Most of these symptoms have also been linked to the male menopause. Strategies for dealing with all these symptoms are discussed on the pages that follow.

hot flashes Often the first sign of perimenopause, these can feel like a creeping, claustrophobic heat radiating from the chest, face, and upper body, lasting for up to several minutes before declining (usually with increased perspiration, especially on face).

night sweats Periods of overheating and profuse sweating during sleep, causing wakefulness and the need to remove bedding to cool the body down.

declining libido Libido may gradually diminish and can be hastened by the discovery intercourse is painful (see next).

painful intercourse As the vaginal wall changes, and arousal can fail to produce sufficient lubrication, sex can become difficult, which can lead to a decrease in desire in itself.

tiredness Tiredness and lack of energy are often reported, although these might be part of a general decline in physical health that can occur in some women at this age, or because of an over-busy lifestyle.

insomnia Women who have previously slept "like a log" report they have trouble getting off to sleep, or wake during the night with their minds racing and can't get back to sleep.

depression Women who have never been prone to depression report unexplained feelings of sadness or misery. Again, some experts believe this isn't a direct medical result of menopause, but a linked reaction to losing fertility and getting older.

irritability and mood swings Many women report a decrease in patience and an increase in irritability and short temper. Well, with so many symptoms to cope with, it is very understandable… but these symptoms might have a hormonal base, similar to the depressed mood many women feel before a period. Mood swings are also common.

joint aches and pains Pain or discomfort, tightness and stiffness in the joints, with no arthritis present, are often reported during menopause and it is thought that these might be linked with hormonal changes altering the make-up of the tissue.

headache or migraine Probably hormonal, as with premenstrual headaches.

poor memory Memory for names, times, and appointments seems to be particularly badly affected during menopause.

coping with menopause

- Remember menopause is not a disease—it is a "rite of passage." Say goodbye to your child-bearing years with a tinge of regret, but also with a sense of looking forward to the future. Many women in their 50s can testify that a zest for life is psychological, not hormonal, and research shows a positive attitude to your life can diminish menopausal symptoms. For ideas on improving the quality of your life, see Chapter 5, Time for Your New Life.

- Freedom from periods and unexpected pregnancy can be a bonus to cherish.

- Much research shows menopausal symptoms become worse when you are under stress. All the stress-reducing tactics outlined on pages 202–3 might help you to cope without recourse to HRT.

- Smoking, alcohol, and caffeine make hot flashes worse, so cut these down or out.

- Reduce the annoyance of hot flashes by taking a hand-held fan plus a small canister of spray water with you in your bag.

- Choose clothes with a low neckline to avoid the claustrophobic feeling that can accompany hot flashes.

- Choose fine-weave clothes in natural fibers— layered in winter—rather than heavy, thick manmade items.

- Acupuncture can help alleviate menopausal symptoms.

- Help prevent osteoporosis by taking 1,500mg a day calcium citrate.

- Fifteen minutes weight training a day (see pages 104–7) can strengthen bones, as well as muscles.

For females, the standard medical treatment for the past several decades has been with hormone replacement therapy (HRT), which has been claimed to be virtually the elixir of life for women over 50. Medics have promoted it as not only a cure for the worst menopausal symptoms, such as hot flashes and decreased libido, but also as a long-term preventive for heart disease and osteoporosis. Many users claimed to feel reinvigorated and sexy, and to have improved skin, hair, and health.

Indeed, HRT using estrogen and progesterone does seem to work well in eliminating hot flashes and, for as long as it is taken, protect against bone loss. (Both flashes and bone loss will reoccur if the HRT is stopped.) How much of the improvement is due to the "placebo" effect is, however, a matter of argument—one controlled trial of more than 16,000 women published in 2003 concluded HRT taken over a year did NOT improve well-being and its effects were largely in the mind.

In recent years, however, HRT has caused great controversy in the medical profession. It cannot be taken by women who already have, or have had, breast or womb cancer. For other women, research shows the combined estrogen/progesterone pill can double the risk of breast cancer—and can also increase the risk of heart disease, stroke, blood clots, and dementia. Because of these scares—and because about 15 percent women experience side effects like bloating, weight gain, breast tenderness, headaches, and nausea when taking HRT—many women have stopped taking it and are keen to try less invasive or more natural alternatives.

other medication

Rather than taking HRT pills, you can use patches, nasal spray, or even implants, all of which can be a better alternative for some. Recent research has determined antidepressant drugs known as selective serotonin reuptake inhibitors (SSRIs), such as paroxetine and venlafaxine, can help reduce flashes and night sweats by up to 70 percent and would, obviously, help depression and anxiety. Raloxifene hydrochloride might help prevent osteo-porosis and might cut the risk of heart disease and stroke, while bisphosphonate can stop bone loss within six months. See your doctor to discuss the pros and cons of these alternatives in your case.

natural alternatives to HRT

The first line of attack is diet, discussed on pages 54–9. A suitable healthy diet can help avoid weight gain and might reduce other symptoms. Research also shows regular exercise is a good way to minimize hot flashes, as well as to control weight and keep fit. Stretching and yoga can help joint aches and pains, while weight-bearing exercise helps maintain bone density. All types of exercise will help in getting better sleep and promote relaxation and better mood—see Chapter 2.

supplements and creams

There is a bewildering range of dietary supplements available claiming to control hot flashes and other symptoms. Most haven't been the subject of clinical trials and so their efficacy is mostly anecdotal. There is additional information on plant estrogens and menopause on pages 56–7. Avoid estrogenic supplements if you have breast cancer.

Red clover—Contains isoflavones (see page 56 and soy below).

Black cohosh—Routinely used in Germany to treat menopausal symptoms and said to be one of the best relievers for flashes and sweating by acting on the hypothalamus to regulate temperature. It can also ease anxiety, insomnia, and mood swings. Currently undergoing large trials to determine safety and validity. One recent research paper using mice found it could speed the spread of breast cancer, while a clinical trial found it had less effect than a placebo. Nevertheless, it has more professional fans than most of the other herbal remedies.

Dong quai—For hormonal imbalance.

Agnus castus (*chaste tree*)—For hormonal imbalance.

Sage—Said to relieve hot flashes by 56 percent in a small trial; might help minimize night sweats.

Soy—High in isoflavones, which might give relief from menopausal symptoms and might help to protect bones, although evidence is conflicting. Might also help protect against heart disease.

Various supplements mixing two or more of these are widely available. Remember even natural remedies may have hidden dangers or side effects.

Progesterone creams (like wild yam) are available via the Internet. Many women find 2–3ml rubbed into fatty skin areas reduces hot flashes, but effectiveness against osteoporosis or cancer isn't clinically proven.

tips for male menopause

In most males, androgens (hormones such as testosterone) drop at about 1 percent per annum after the 30s, rather than there being an 80 percent drop within a few short years, as is the case with the female menopause. However, about 5 percent of men suffer androgen deficiency syndrome, when the male hormone replacement therapy (TRT) might be useful.

There is evidence that implants are more effective than testosterone pills, which, for men experiencing the normal gradual drop in hormones, have not proved effective in improving sexual function. For erection problems, Viagra is a better bet for most. For more information on improving libido in mid life, see Libido on pages 178–83. Testosterone has not been shown to improve bone density in men.

Whether the decline in androgen levels is sharp or more gradual, a number of men report hot flashes during midlife. There is a definite link—when men suffering from prostate cancer have androgen deprivation as part of their therapy, 80 percent suffer from hot flashes and sleep disturbance.

Factors which might speed the reduction of testosterone levels in men include stress, weight gain, high alcohol intake, and lack of exercise. So the moral seems to be—lead a healthy life with plenty of activity and relaxation.

- Avoid a Body Mass Index (BMI) over 27 or 28.

- Slow down your pace of work to match your energy levels.

- Do daily regular aerobic exercises, such as walking, and weight-bearing exercise, such as weightlifting.

- Have no more than two glasses of alcohol a day and take two days off from drinking a week.

- Enjoy life.

well-being and **libido**

There really is no standard for libido. It is totally subjective and so all that matters is that you—and your partner—are happy with what you have. One thing is for certain—you don't have to have sex to make love. Here we consider the difference between sex and lovemaking, and look at all the ways that libido can be boosted, if you feel that's what you need.

The first thing you should know about libido is the statistics you read in the papers and magazines about how often other people have sex rarely paint an accurate picture. The fact is more people lie about sex than about any other human function. Everyone wants others to think they have sex more often than they do.

lies, damn lies, and statistics

So any statistician hoping to get the truth is wasting his or her time. For example, a recent study from the National Opinion Research Center, at Chicago University, investigating sexual habits in people over 50, found there was only a marginal decline in the amount of sexual activity (five times a month) compared with young adults (six or seven times a month). In another study, 90 percent of men aged 80 or over said they were still sexually active. This might, of course, all be accurate—but it might not. The clinical fact is physical sex drive declines with age because, in midlife and old age, levels of the sex hormones decline.

does declining libido matter?

When it comes to sex, the only thing that really matters is whether or not you are happy with your situation. There is evidence that a reasonably high percentage of long- (and presumably fairly happily) married couples in midlife don't have sex at all, and are perfectly satisfied. Other single people (perhaps divorced or widowed) give up sex and are happy to remain celibate. Problems only arise when one or other partner is unhappy with their sex life, or when a single or newly divorced person finds they can't get an erection, or can't face sex with someone even if attracted to them. Seek help from a doctor if you think you or your partner might have a medical problem affecting your sex life. Many problems can be easily resolved.

Even if you can't have intercourse every night—or every month—what you CAN do is make love. Kissing, cuddling, and snuggling up together are all as important—or more important—than actual sex.

the trouble with sex ...

If you are unhappy with the quality of your own libido, that of your partner, or your sex life in general, there is plenty that can be done to improve matters. We look at the most common reasons why your sex life can take a downturn in midlife, and discuss how you might deal with them ...

the natural decline of sex hormones

As we saw in the last chapter on menopause and andropause, midlife is a time when the sexual hormone levels can drop rapidly— certainly for women, while for many men, it is a more gentle decline, the cumulative effect of which becomes noticeable around fifty. A drop in these hormones is a major reason for a lessening of desire in both sexes and what is sometimes coyly termed a "decline in sexual performance" in men.

Conventional hormone replacement therapy can improve libido in women, while TRT (male HRT, using testosterone) can have a similar effect for men, and new research says testosterone can also be used to enhance enjoyment of sex by women.

All hormonal treatments are available in pill, patch, injection, implant, and other forms—see your doctor for advice. Not everyone, however, wants to try drug therapy, and for many people a decline in the regularity or urgency of sex can be acceptable ... it is the body telling us that our child-bearing years are coming to a natural end. That said, one recent report finds 50 percent males aged 70 are still fully potent, (in other words, able to get and maintain erection and achieve ejaculation,) and for many women, having a man take longer is actually a bonus. For both sexes, greater attention to foreplay and "taking your time" can more than make up for any shortfalls in hormones.

the natural aging process Several

factors have a bearing on sexual function as we age. In men, nerve impulses slow down, which decreases genital sensitivity, and the arteries in the penis are less able to maintain the blood pressure necessary for an erection, which can cause erectile dysfunction (see also Poor health, Psychological factors, and Lifestyle opposite and page 182). Viagra and the new rash of similar drugs are designed to overcome erectile problems by increasing blood flow to the penis, and these are the best solution for most older men. Other variations on the theme are coming along, too—there are creams that claim to work more quickly than sidenafil (Viagra's active agent). Ask your doctor for advice. Nonchemical ways to improve potency include the natural herbs gingko biloba, ginseng, and tribulus terrestrus.

For women, vaginal lubrication can be a problem and, as in men, a decline in blood circulation can mean less sensitivity in the area. The walls of the vagina also become thinner and less elastic and this can make sexual intercourse difficult and cause tearing of the vaginal lining and/or pain. A doctor can prescribe jelly for simple lubrication, or estrogen-containing creams. There is also a device approved by the US Food and Drug Administration (US FDA) called the Eros CTD, a vacuum instrument that improves blood flow to the vaginal area.

Herbs that can help females include dong quai, said to improve vaginal lubrication; aloe vera juice, and damiana, said to increase sex drive, while vitamins C and E can help maintain vaginal tissue.

For both sexes, "use it or lose it" is a good maxim—research shows regular sex, three times a week for preference—does keep the sexual organs working better, no matter your age, with foreplay of extreme importance for both sexes. Daily pelvic floor squeezing for women also helps maintain muscle tone in the vaginal area, while aerobic exercise improves circulation (including to the penis) for men.

poor health Research has found, hardly

surprisingly, that in mid- and old age it is those who retain good health who are most likely to continue with an active sex life, while people in poor health are most likely to be celibate. Diabetes and athero-sclerosis (hardening of the arteries) are both known to have an effect on erectile function in men. (See also Drugs, Lifestyle, and Psychological factors).

Likewise, a good sex life improves your health. Sex improves the circulation, can lower blood levels of "bad" cholesterol, cause relaxation hormones to be released to relieve stress, release natural pain-killing endorphins, and keep the prostate healthy.

drugs It is estimated 25 percent of all male

impotence is induced by prescription or over-the-counter drugs. Known culprits include some types of medication for high blood pressure, nonsteroidal antiinflammatory drugs, tranquilizers, antihistamines, and many antidepressants, although depression itself can cause impotence—see Psychological Factors—so these latter statistics might be suspect. Recreational drugs, like cannabis, can also reduce libido, as can alcohol and tobacco (see Lifestyle).

psychological factors Stress, anxiety,

fatigue, and, most of all, depression can contribute to libido loss in both sexes and impotence in men. About 90 percent depressed men suffer some degree of impotence. The answer is to treat these psychological causes—which can be nothing to do with sex, but are often related to problems at work or in other areas of home and family life.

lifestyle A well-balanced lifestyle can boost sexual performance and libido. At least in part, this means leading a healthy day-to-day life, with moderation in most things being the key. Keep alcohol intake low. Even fairly moderate amounts of alcohol can cause "brewer's droop" at any age, and can dull the nerves to the female sex organs, too. Nicotine can also anaesthetize the sex organs. Lack of regular exercise appears to be directly linked to poor sexual function, and you need to do not only aerobic exercise to increase circulation, but also loosening and stretching exercises, particularly of the neck and shoulders. Tight neck muscles can restrict the circulation around the head and neck and might impede the work of the hypothalamus, which regulates all hormonal functions.

A good diet is very important. Several of the foods in The Top 20 Foods for Antiaging on pages 20–3 have a good effect on your libido—particularly those high in antioxidants, and a generally healthy diet will boost health (see Poor health). The classic libidinous foods, oysters, are rich in zinc, but if you don't happen to like them, plenty of nuts, seeds, whole grains, other seafood, and leafy greens—all good sources of the mineral—will do the trick.

emotional baggage Even if your
hormones are still raging, you both look great and you still want sex, sometimes years of builtup negative emotions directed at your partner can dull libido so much you just can't do it with that person any more. Women seem more prone to sexual turn-off because of psychological factors, but they can easily affect men, too.

Research shows anger is the emotion most likely to diminish desire for your partner—resentment, frustration, fear, unspoken issues. If the cause(s) of these feelings can be resolved, sex life can often be restored, too. Counseling together might be an idea.

the question of familiarity There has been recent debate on the fact that lessening desire for the same person over time is very normal and natural. When someone is new and exciting, sex is also new and exciting. If, though, you've lived with someone for twenty, thirty, or forty years—and know every inch of their anatomy and their habits—excitement hardly comes into it. If you feel you or your partner might simply be feeling bored with sex, the most tried and tested methods of getting that frisson back is either to use what are now termed "sex toys" (widely available in sex stores or on the Internet) or to try sex videos/manuals, or any other erotica, to get aroused together.

Of course, perhaps your partner is no longer attracted to you. Blunt as this sounds, you might not be getting sex from your partner because he or she just doesn't fancy the way you look any more. Visual appeal is a huge part of sexual attraction for most of us. Not just for sex appeal, but also for our well-being and confidence, it is important not to "let yourself go." Other sections of this book aim to help you stay looking really good (Exercise, Looks)—and not just "for your age" but really good, period. If it is you who no longer desires your partner, then encouragement for them to scrub up and shape up is called for.

the reproductive years are over
The main point of sex is to procreate the human race. Whoever invented it made it so good when we are young because that is when we are fertile. Obviously there are women and men in their midlife who still have children—and men can be fertile into their 80s—but once the reproductive years are at an end the original motivation for sex is no longer be there. Although few people admit it, for a lot of women in particular, sex is more about having babies than about pleasure. There are, no doubt, many thousands of men in their 40s and 50s wondering why their wives no longer want sex, and this might be the simple answer. This is something that needs discussing, not ignoring.

simple ways to boost your libido

- **don't worry about what you think others do** Just think about what you (and your partner) want to do. Your sex life is not a competition. Massage each other or just cuddle—sex might follow naturally if you stop worrying.

- **talk to your partner** Not everyone can feel like sex all the time. Keep up good communication so you can explain, without loss of face or rancor on their part, when you feel like it and when you don't. Expect the same of them. Knowing you can both do this makes sex very much better when you do do it.

- **enjoy life** Research shows people who lead an interesting life, have fun, and regularly circulate with new people find their sex lives improve.

- **use it so you don't lose it** Research shows people who have sex regularly find it easier and more pleasurable than those who only have it occasionally. Even if at first you find it a bit of a "chore," libido DOES return the more often you have sex, and for women, vaginal lubrication improves, too.

- **keep an open mind** Many people give up on sex because they feel it isn't "normal" to want it as they get older. A positive attitude can work wonders.

- **look at the positives of changing sexual performance or appetite** For example, as men get older they might not be able to have an orgasm six times a night, but they can "keep going for longer" each time they do have sex.

- **a new relationship**—or reworking the boundaries of an old one—can reawaken libido. Time apart from a long-term partner might do the trick.

- **get something new into your sex life** While I abhor advice to women to wear frilly pants around the house and dress up in silk stockings and little else to greet your partner as he arrives home (it's more likely to embarrass or frighten the guy), a bit of sexual titillation is always a good idea... sexy underwear in the bedroom, a sex manual, a soft-porn DVD ... that kind of thing.

- **people in good health enjoy sex more** Eat well, exercise regularly, and avoid too much alcohol, cigarettes, or recreational drugs, all of which affect libido and sexual functioning.

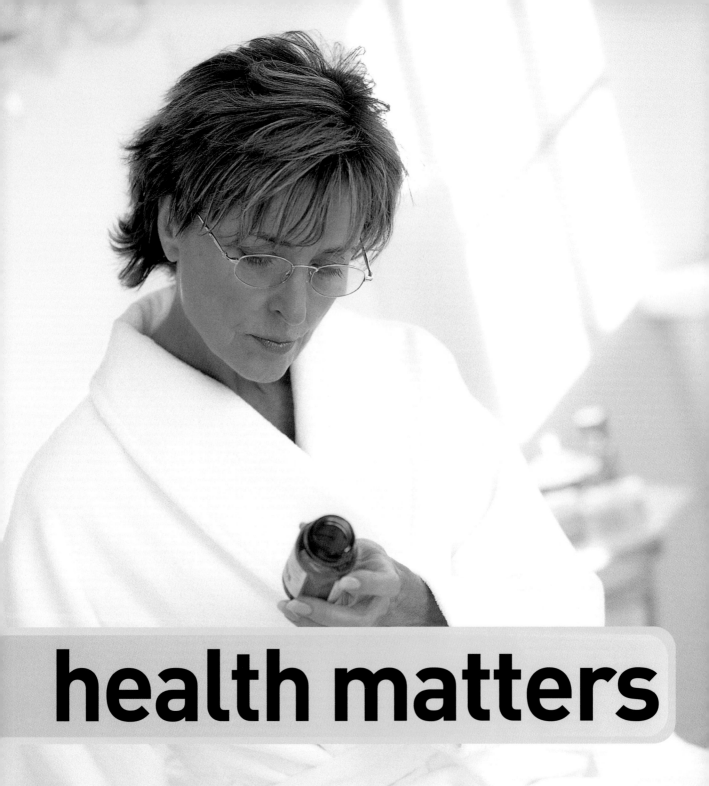

health matters

To enjoy your life you need a certain standard of health—in other words, the best health you can have given your circumstances and what has gone before. This chapter aims to help you deal with the most common health problems of midlife.

As you read through this section you might feel you suffer from more than your fair share of the complaints and illnesses that it describes. Even if you have not felt you were in blooming good health in recent years, it is surprising what can be achieved with even minimal attention to yourself and/or lifestyle changes.

If you are in good shape, however, it is still important to take care of yourself as a preventive measure … for good health is even more vital as you get older. It is your key to independence and the single most wished-for factor when people are asked what they want for their old age.

We will look at the most common syndrome associated with midlife, "tired all the time," and the associated complaints of lethargy and lack of energy. These syndromes might have both physical and psychological causes, all of which we discuss.

Of course, if you are tired, you might have insomnia. Nearly everyone in midlife suffers from this at least some of the time and, in the long term, it can have a drastic effect on your life and that of those close to you. The tips that I give are those that have worked best for others.

The second most common group of complaints in midlife is "aches and pains"—whether from arthritis or other musculoskeletal problems. If you are forced to spend much of the day being painfully aware of your body, this dominates everything. There is, however, much you can do to improve the situation.

It is said 65 percent of over-40s have what they consider to be a poor digestive system, complaining most frequently of (in descending order) heartburn, bloating, irritable bowel, and constipation … We look at what can be done, and discuss the relevance of overindulgence in alcohol, tobacco, and recreational drugs.

Two-thirds of us will eventually get some form of cancer or heart disease … we examine how you can help beat the odds and keep at bay these potential killers—as well as the other big disease of middle age, diabetes.

Lastly, a healthy body needs a healthy mind, so if anxiety, stress, depression, or poor memory drag you down, even if only occasionally, we have some solutions with which to end the section.

tiredness and lethargy If you are physically and mentally shattered or lacking in energy for much of your day, the problem needs resolving—"tired all the time" is a growing problem and, for many, it first occurs in midlife.

the many causes of tiredness

Trying to pinpoint exactly what is causing your feelings of tiredness might not be simple, as there are many possible explanations. Here are the main potential causes.

Being female! Women are more prone to tiredness than men, according to a Scottish study (by men!) published in the *British Medical Journal*. This is thought to be because women are more conditioned to do multitasking, rather than because they are in any way the "weaker sex." So if you are female, try to make a special effort to pace yourself, don't ignore the need for a rest now and then, and get enough sleep. If you have PMS or are experiencing menopause, you are even more likely to feel tired because, due to hormonal changes, fatigue is a common complaint at both these times. Good diet and enough exercise will help.

Depression People with a history of depression are much more likely to report feeling tired. So if you think your tiredness might have psychological origins, see your doctor and/or a therapist for help, and see also Mind Matters (page 198). If your depression is "circumstantial"—in other words, there are specific factors that are bringing you down, then Chapter 5 might help.

Emotional stress Even if you aren't depressed, emotional strain can bring you down, especially in the long term. Permanent overwork, too many things to juggle, relationship problems, family troubles … all these can increase tiredness. Relaxation techniques and a conscious effort to build time for yourself are important.

Physical stress When your body is under stress it is normal for it to react by feeling tired. Stress of the kind that makes you have symptoms of nervousness or anxiety (palpitations, dry mouth, perspiration, for example) causes the release of adrenaline and if this is prolonged it literally wears you out. Get regular daily exercise, and see pages 202–3 for dealing with stress.

Medical conditions Illness is another stress for the body—coping with serious illness in the short term (a bad bout of flu) or in the long term can make you tired—you need to make sure to give yourself time to "be ill" and time to recover. Several medical conditions are recognized as having tiredness as one of their symptoms. These include Epstein Barr (glandular fever), flu and bronchitis, anemia, cancer, diabetes, hypothyroidism, multiple sclerosis, liver disease, heart, and lung disease. They also include disorders such as sleep apnea and chronic fatigue syndrome. See your doctor if you feel a medical condition could be causing your tiredness.

Lack of rest Obvious as it sounds, one common cause of tiredness and lack of energy is "overdoing it." If you are on the go all day every day, you are going to feel tired some of the time. It isn't always necessary to be busy sixteen hours a day (see Chapter 5).

Too much rest Ah! But too much rest can also make you feel tired—probably by reducing the amount of oxygen that gets to the brain. For more on this, see pages 188–9.

Poor quality of sleep Even if you get seven or eight hours in bed, you can be tired because of poor sleep patterns or even sleep apnea. See overleaf.

Poor exercise and lifestyle habits Too little exercise can make you feel tired and reduce your body's capacity to deal with a busy life. Exercise is one of the best "cures" for daytime tiredness and lack of energy, as long as it is moderate (such as walking) rather than hard/vigorous. In the short term, the increase in blood circulation—and, therefore, available oxygen—has a regenerating effect on the brain, which is the seat of much fatigue. In the long term, increased fitness can help you keep going for longer.

Poor diet Can induce tiredness by not providing enough of the energy-converting vitamins and other nutrients. Drastic dieting can also mean there aren't enough calories available to provide energy.

ideas for boosting energy levels and banishing tiredness

- **eat a balanced breakfast** to sustain you through the morning and have a high-protein lunch containing only small amounts of good-quality carbs. A lunch high in carbs, especially those such as white bread or white pasta, will make you feel tired in the afternoon as they encourage production of sleep-inducing hormones.

- **get as much fresh air as you can** Try to work in a room where you can have the window open; and sleep with the window ajar. Stale air makes you feel stagnant.

- **keep the heat down low** If your brain is too warm, you will soon feel tired and your brain will slow down.

- **avoid sugary drinks and snacks** for energy during the day. The boost they give will be short-term, and within an hour you'll feel more tired than ever. Instead have small amounts of lean protein, like yogurt or nuts and seeds.

- **for an instant reviver**, do 1 minute's skipping or marching on the spot, with arms moving, or running up and down stairs. This increases circulation and carries oxygen to the brain.

- **take a 5-minute siesta** Research shows this fits in with the body's circadian rhythms and people who take a nap, say, midafternoon, perform better for the rest of the day than people who don't.

- **several supplements** are claimed to help improve energy levels. Coenzyme Q10 is particularly good for improving stamina for exercise. Acetyl-l-carnitine and alpha lipoic acid used together may increase energy by boosting mitochondria, the internal combustion engine of cells. Iron pills may help, even if you are not anaemic.

- **drink 2 quarts fluids a day** – preferably water. Your brain needs to be only 3 percent dehydrated to affect mental and physical performance considerably.

aches and pains Joint, muscular, and other aches and pains
can cause much misery in midlife, but there is plenty you can do to ease these problems.

arthritis

The word "arthritis" means damage to, or disease of, the joints. There two most common types are osteo-arthritis, and rheumatoid arthritis.

Osteoarthritis affects about 80 percent people over 50 to some degree and is sometimes called "wear and tear," because the cartilage cushioning the joints thins and can wear out completely. This causes pain, stiffness, and sometimes swelling, as well as other changes in the joint, and can limit range of movement. It's common in the knees, hips, hands, and spine, and is not usually associated with redness and heat in the area.

Obesity can put extra strain on the lower joints and make arthritis worse. While medical treatment is usually confined to painkillers or nonsteroidal antiinflammatory drugs (NSAIDs)—and sometimes, eventually, joint replacement—there is much you can do to help minimize the negative side effects of arthritis (see the panel opposite).

Rheumatoid arthritis is an inflammatory disease occurring more often in women than in men, and more frequently in younger adults than osteoarthritis, often beginning with weakness and pain in the hands. Although there is a theory that an infection can be the cause, this hasn't been proved. The disease can be unpredictable, with periods of remission, but eventually joints may become swollen, red, and inflamed. Other symptoms can include tiredness, loss of weight, feeling unwell, fever, and night sweats, and even a rash or mouth ulcers. Many of the helpful hints for osteoarthritis are also useful (see opposite).

fibromyalgia

This painful condition of the muscles, tendons, and/or ligaments, rather than in the joints, tends to hit about the late 40s, and only one in ten sufferers is male. There might be multiple sore points around the body—often in the shoulders, outer elbows, or chest.

Sufferers often sleep badly and, conversely, can develop fibromyalgia if they have chronic insomnia. The condition is also linked with depression, stress, and trauma, and there is no diagnostic test as it is a descriptive term rather than a medical condition. Fibromyalgia can spontaneously get better, and can sometimes be improved with regular moderate exercise. Good news is sufferers are not at higher risk of arthritis. (See opposite for additional tips.)

polymyalgia rheumatica (PMR)

This is a disease that can be diagnosed by a blood test and tends to affect about four in every thousand people over 50. The cause is unknown, but symptoms are pain and stiffness (worse in the mornings), often around the shoulders and thighs, and perhaps feeling unwell and tired. There can also be inflammation in the arteries around the temple in severe cases. Treatment is usually steroids, which might be needed for several years—the condition can often be cured, but can be almost permanent in some. All the other aches and pains described above can be mistaken for PMR, so diagnosis is important.

headaches

There are very many possible causes of headache, including hormonal changes, stress, dehydration, diet, illness (such as an infection or fever). Most headaches are short-lived and can be controlled with over-the-counter painkillers—but don't rely on these, as research shows that they can actually, with overuse, make headaches worse. Migraine headaches can often be improved with feverfew tincture or tablets. If prone to frequent unexplained headaches it is a good idea to see your doctor.

other aches and pains

"Rheumatism" is a blanket expression for unexplained aches and pains around the joints. "Tennis elbow" and "housemaid's knee" are examples of rheumatism.

beating arthritis and other aches and pains

Use the tips that are most appropriate to your case—
and see your doctor for additional advice.

- **special diet** Many words have been written about special exclusion diets to help arthritis, but the Arthritis Foundation says that, other than maintaining a healthy weight and eating a balanced diet, there is rarely any benefit in eating a special diet. "You should be suspicious of any diet that claims to treat or cure arthritis. If such a diet existed, you can be sure your doctor would know about it and recommend the diet to you." Foods most often claimed to make arthritis worse are citrus fruits, potatoes, tomatoes, eggplants, and bell peppers, coffee, and red wine. Meat might also be a trigger for rheumatoid arthritis, according to one 2000 study found. Research published in late 2003 also shows meat contains a type of molecule the tissues can absorb and which might cause inflammation.

- **the omega-3 oils in oily fish** and cod liver oil have been proved to be helpful in relieving the pain and disability of arthritis. If you don't enjoy oily fish, take fish oil supplements instead—1,000mg a day is normal.

- **keep your body weight down**—vital for helping osteoarthritis.

- **several supplements** might help the pain and stiffness of arthritis and other musculoskeletal complaints. These include bromelian, an enzyme found in pineapples; the spices ginger and turmeric; glucosamine, which can help form joint cartilage; chondroitin, which works well together with glucosamine to keep the joints healthy; and methyl sulphonyl methane (MSM), which is another component of cartilage structure. Collagen supplements can stimulate the growth of new cartilage and help pain, while the herbs nettles, rue, and boswellian are said to be antiinflammatory. Green-lipped mussels and devil's claw might also work for some. For tight muscles and stiffness, the mineral magnesium can act as a relaxer.

- **regular gentle-to-moderate exercise** works to maintain joint mobility—yoga, stretching, and swimming are all ideal. All joints should be put through their full range of movement once a day, to prevent them stiffening.

- **a heat pad** placed on the site of pain can help, as can a cold pad.

the digestive system

When we are young, the digestive system can often take a great deal of abuse or be ignored and still behave in an impeccable manner. As we get older, however, this is no longer the case. The gut needs a lot of looking after! So, starting from the top ...

heartburn/indigestion

Heartburn—pain behind the breastbone, often radiating to neck and arm, caused by stomach acids rising into the gullet—is frequently mistaken for a heart attack, while dyspepsia, or indigestion, refers to general pain and discomfort in the abdominal area and chest.

Heartburn is most frequently caused by overweight, eating large meals, bending over, or smoking. Younger women find it common during pregnancy. Frequent heartburn can be a sign of hiatus hernia and you should get it checked by your doctor.

Dyspepsia can be caused by irritation of the stomach lining and/or duodenum, which can be due to overeating, anxiety, or certain foods or drinks—fatty foods, spices, coffee, and alcohol are the most common. Some drugs can also irritate the stomach and cause ulcers, notably aspirin and some nonsteroidal antiinflammatory drugs (NSAIDS).

CURES: Over-the-counter antacid remedies might work, but shouldn't be relied on too much. Best advice? Stop smoking, maintain a suitable weight, eat small frequent meals, avoid foods and/or drinks you know trigger attacks, and see your doctor to check if other problems, such as peptic ulcer, are the cause.

bloating

The most common cause of bloating is a meal rich in carbohydrates, particularly refined white carbs based on grains—white bread, white pasta, cakes, or cookies. Carbs act like blotting paper to retain liquid in the body. A high-salt snack or meal has a similar effect—the body retains fluid to try to dilute the salt to a reasonable level, as high sodium concentrations can be dangerous. Thirdly, intestinal wind (gas) can cause bloating—typical causes of a gassy stomach are legumes (beans, chickpeas, lentils), onions, cabbage and other brassicas, wheat, and dried fruit. All these foods are "good for you," so rather than eliminating them, eat them well cooked, finely chopped or puréed, in small amounts. Women

preperiod or during menopause can be more prone to bloating—fresh fruit, salads, and lean protein should not produce this effect. In general, chew food thoroughly, eat little and often, and try to relax while eating ... stressful meals can cause bloating.

irritable bowel syndrome (IBS)

It is estimated 20 percent of the American adult population—and twice as many women as men—suffer from IBS, which is not a disease, but a set of symptoms that can vary from person to person, and can come and go. The most common are abdominal cramps and pain, bloating, flatulence, and either loose bowels or constipation, perhaps alternating.

There are links between the onset of IBS and stress, and it can be triggered by illness, or can be caused by food intolerance. Wheat and dairy products are the two most common allergens for IBS sufferers and, indeed, the symptoms are similar to those of lactose intolerance (inability to digest the sugars in milk products). A course of probiotics (available from pharmacies and health food stores—only buy if kept in the refrigerator) can also help relieve IBS by colonizing the gut with gut-friendly bacteria.

Relaxation and cognitive behavior therapy seem to improve symptoms by up to 70 percent, while a basic elimination diet can find out if you are intolerant of any food(s). In general, a healthy diet and lifestyle, including regular exercise can help.

constipation

One in six people—most often women—suffer from constipation, and many of these are aged over 50. Usually the problem can be fairly easily overcome with correct diet and exercise (see 10 Ways to Keep Regular, opposite). This is the most sensible way to treat it rather than resorting to laxatives, which can upset the natural balance of the intestines and bowel. The body can also become used to them, so you need more and more for them to work.

ways to keep regular

- **include high-fiber foods** at every meal, with a balance of both soluble and insoluble fiber.

- **find insoluble fiber in** whole-grain bread, cereals, brown rice, and whole-wheat pasta; in leafy green vegetables, nuts, and seeds; and in reasonable quantities in other vegetables, fruit, and legumes.

- **find soluble fiber in** most fresh and dried fruits, especially citrus fruits, apples, mangoes; in legumes; and also in reasonable quantities in oats, barley, and rye.

- **aim for at least 6g of total fiber per meal**—most food packaging carry fiber information. If already constipated, aim for 8g fiber per meal.

- **eat 7 portions of fruit and vegetables a day**, and eat whole fruit rather than fruit juice, which has the fiber removed.

- **drink 2 quarts liquids a day** and aim for at least half of this to be water. Without enough liquid, high-fiber foods cannot do their job of increasing the bulk of stools and making them pass easily through the gut.

- **prunes and rhubarb** contain compounds that help ease constipation, so they should be included in your diet a few times a week.

- **go for natural "health-food" remedies** rather than harsh laxatives from a pharmacist. Rosehip syrup, olive oil, honey, licorice, molasses, psyllium seed, and curry spices all have a laxative effect.

- **a course of probiotics will also help**—these are natural gut bacteria that seem to have a laxative effect for most people.

- **do regular daily exercise**—both aerobic exercise, such as brisk walking, and other exercise, such as toning or weight training, will help stimulate the gut into action.

the big three
Heart disease, cancer, and diabetes are the three diseases most likely to affect people in midlife. Here we look at the implications...

heart disease

Cardiovascular disease (CVD—an umbrella term that includes high blood pressure, heart attack, angina, congestive heart failure, stroke, and congenital heart defects) is the single largest cause of American deaths. In 2001, CVD killed 931,000 Americans, of which about 499,000 were women. (This compares to 266,700 women who died from all forms of cancer.) CVD is most likely to hit men over 45 and women over 55 – and the major risk factors, other than genetics, stem from your choice of lifestyle.

A diet for a healthy heart needs to be low in saturated fat – recent research shows that even an excess 100g of saturates a week can increase women's risk of dying from heart disease by nearly 38 percent. Monounsaturated fats, such as olive oil, and omega-3 fats from oily fish can, on the other hand, protect the heart. Leafy vegetables (rich in B vitamins B_6, B_{12}, and folate to help prevent high homocysteine levels in the blood, which can be a significant factor in CVD), all fruit and vegetables, nuts, garlic, legumes, soy, and red wine, and the plant chemicals they contain, are all linked with a healthy heart (see Chapter 1).

Lack of exercise is another major factor. The American Heart Association says that even moderate-level exercise will often help lower your risk of heart disease. In fact, studies show that being physically fit lowers heart disease risk, even in people who have other health problems, such as high blood pressure. See Chapter 2 for more information.

Good diet and exercise will help prevent overweight or obesity, which are also high risk factors, and they will also help prevent high blood pressure and a poor blood-fats profile (high in LDL cholesterol, homocysteine, and triglycerides), which are both risk factors for CVD.

A high percentage of heart deaths are due to tobacco smoking, which increases the blood's capacity to clot, and drugs, such as cocaine that can also cause heart failure. Alcohol is fine for most people in small amounts (1 to 2 glasses a day have a beneficial effect on the heart for people in midlife and later), but heavy and binge drinking are linked with heart attacks.

Stress can also cause CVD—a study of over 3,000 adults showed a definite link between long-term anger, anxiety, impatience, and stress with increased blood pressure and, therefore, heart disease. Overwork really can kill—working 60 hours a week doubles the risk of a coronary. On the other hand, getting enough sleep and laughter, and antistress devices, like stroking pets, can reduce blood pressure and dangerous blood fats.

women and heart disease

The general feeling is that women's risk of CVD has increased in recent years because of their increasingly hectic and unhealthy lifestyles. While it is thought the hormone estrogen offers women protection against heart disease until after menopause, increased levels of stress, smoking, and alcohol intake are canceling out this protective factor. Recently it has also been found that HRT doesn't offer significant protection against heart disease during or after menopause.

cancer

In 2005, it is estimated 1.3 million Americans will be diagnosed with cancer, and 570,000 will die from one form or another of the disease. Lung cancer is the top killer. Up to 70 percent of all cancers could be prevented with lifestyle changes. Smoking accounts for 30 percent, while diet is thought to cause 35 percent.

heart facts ● Aspirin offers double protection against heart disease, by helping prevent blood clots from forming and by stopping inflammation in the arteries. ● Women with diabetes are five times as likely to have heart disease as nondiabetics—the relative risk for diabetic men is lower.

The World Health Organization's World Cancer Report (2003) said that cancer-inducing lifestyle factors include alcohol intake, lack of exercise, obesity, and low intake of fruit and vegetables. Other probable causes include infectious diseases, a negative outlook, which can compromise the immune system, and exposure to heavy metals in the atmosphere and food.

In midlife, three of the most common cancers are of the lung, breast, and prostate. Lung cancer is mainly caused by tobacco smoking or passive smoking and it is never too late to give up—your risk of getting cancer begins to reduce almost immediately after you stop, and continues to reduce until after fifteen years your risk is no greater than that of someone who has never smoked. A diet rich in fruit and vegetables might help to protect against lung cancer, and an American study found selenium supplementation caused a 50 percent drop in deaths from lung cancer. Selenium is found in high quantities in Brazil nuts. (See Chapter 1.)

Breast cancer causes one-third of all female cancers, and is the second-leading cause of cancer deaths. Death rates, however, are declining with screening and treatment advances. Two main risk factors are obesity, which increases circulating estrogens, and high alcohol intake, while HRT doubles the risk. There might be a link with the trend to have fewer babies, as exposure to high estrogen levels are reduced with pregnancy.

A healthy diet, low in saturated fat, and with a high content of plant foods, including soy, no more than two alcoholic drinks daily, exercise, and relaxation might help prevent breast cancer.

diabetes

Type-2 diabetes, and its frequent precursor, insulin resistance (caused by a diet high in simple carbohydrates, sugar and calories), are the modern "plagues." Diabetes affects 18.2 million people in the United States, most in middle age and above. In the long term, it can cause heart disease, blindness and death. Lifestyle is a very important factor in minimizing the risk of diabetes, weight control being the most obvious. A BMI above 26 in middle-aged men trebles the risk, while one over 30 increases risk by a factor of nine (more if surplus weight is carried, mostly around the waist). Again the prescription is exercise, watching calories, fat, and sugar intake, and eating plenty of fruit, veg, fish, and legumes.

prostate cancer

Prostate cancer is the second most common cancer for American males. The American Cancer Society estimates one in six men get it, but only one in thirty-three will die from it, and that rate is declining. Diet is important in prevention or containing the disease.

- Lycopene, the antioxidant phytochemical found in highest quantities in tomatoes (absorbed best when the tomatoes are cooked) can cut the risk by a third, and onions and onion family members, such as leeks and garlic, might also be protective.

- Broccoli, Brussels sprouts, and other leafy greens contain phytochemicals called indoles that suppress prostate cancer growth by inhibiting hormones that can provoke it.

- Supplements of the mineral selenium over time also reduce the risk of developing the disease.

- It might also be wise to keep animal fat intake low, eat only moderate amounts of dairy produce, and avoid smoked, cured, and charred foods.

- Other lifestyle factors that might minimize the risk include frequent sexual intercourse, which helps to clear cancer-causing chemicals via the semen, and moderate intake of red wine. It is thought the phenols it contains inhibit the growth of prostate cancer cells.

- Many men are now being offered female HRT patches to reduce testosterone production—which can encourage the growth of the cancer cells.

alcohol and drugs Alcohol ... cigarettes ... cannabis ... more than
90 percent of us rely on—or use frequently—at least one addictive substance to help us through life.

alcohol

It is estimated one tenth of American adults suffer from an alcohol or drug use disorder, or both.

In midlife, alcohol tends to be a fixed factor in most people's lives, having been there for perhaps thirty or forty years. Although research shows few people admit that their alcohol intake gives them cause for concern, in fact, many people would prefer to be less beholden to the "cup that cheers."

It is true that there are a few benefits to be gained from moderate alcohol intake. The list – often cited as reason enough to carry on drinking – includes protection from heart attack, dementia, stroke, and viral infections (particularly with moderate intake of red wine). It is thought that the plant chemicals such as polyphenols that alcoholic drinks often contain might have an antioxidant effect.

According to research, however, drinking in moderation is three times as beneficial for men as for women, and the protective effects of alcohol are more likely to benefit men over the age of 55 and women over 65. The American Heart Association, however, advises persons with high blood pressure to avoid alcohol.

The negative aspects of alcohol consumption over the recommended limit of one drink or less a day include increased risk of high blood pressure and cardiovascular disease for heavy drinkers, of liver disease that can lead to cirrhosis, of some cancers (in women, there is a 6 percent increase in risk of breast cancer for every extra alcohol drink consumed a day), of ulcers, gastritis, pancreatitis, gout, and memory loss…. and, of course, weight gain. Half a bottle of wine a day contains about 300 calories, which could put 32 pounds fat on you in the course of a year if in addition to your normal energy requirements.

High alcohol intake can also affect eyesight and cause gum infections, dehydration, palpitations, muscular pains, and accidents around the home and while driving, and is linked with insomnia, increased divorce, unreliability at work, and depression. Plus you get hangovers. Makes you think, doesn't it? Use the tips here to cut down to a safe level. See pages 236–7 for contacts.

tobacco and drugs

The potential dangers of tobacco are well documented— it is the cause of the majority of cases of lung cancer and is one of the major contributors to heart disease and stroke. Despite this, if you have smoked for many years, giving up in midlife isn't easy.

The best course of action is to see your doctor, who might recommend a variety of nicotine replacement therapy (NRT) or Zyban—trials show smokers are twice as likely to succeed in giving up if they use these methods. Willpower alone is often not enough, but it can be done. Use some of the tactics described for reducing alcohol intake.

If you do manage to give up, within 20 minutes of your last cigarette, blood pressure drops, within 8 hours your oxygen blood levels improve, within two days your taste buds begin to return, then lung capacity improves. In five years, your risk of dying is half of what it would have been if you had continued smoking. Smokers can reduce the risks and improve the health of their lungs by eating a healthy diet high in fish and fish oils and in fruit and vegetables, which are rich in antioxidants, especially vitamin C.

Ex-smokers tend to put on about 20 pounds after quitting—this is partly because of the rebirth of the taste buds, partly because snacking is used to replace the act of lighting a cigarette, and partly because nicotine raises the metabolic rate. Being a few pounds heavier is acceptable, healthwise, as a swap for giving up, but you can limit weight gain by eating sensibly and doing plenty of exercise. (See Chapters 1 and 2.)

Cannabis and other so-called "recreational drugs" are a common part of the social scene for young adults—and there are plenty of people in their 50s and 60s who have been using drugs since the '60s and '70s. In the long term, doctors now believe cannabis smoking is as dangerous as nicotine, and is also linked with an increased risk of mental illness and memory problems. The relaxing effects contribute after prolonged use to a "laid-back" mentality, where ideas are not carried through and motivation is lacking. In other words, if you want to make the most of your new midlife, cannabis is not really a friend. Take note of the tips given for cutting back on alcohol and cigarettes.

cutting down on alcohol

- Write a list of all the reasons you want to cut down or give up.

- Work out how much you are spending on alcohol a week or a year and decide on something you would really like to do with that money instead. For instance, $50 a week translates to a really good vacation or a weekly massage.

- Work out how much time you spend choosing alcohol and drinking it, and think of what you could do with that time instead. An hour a day equates to a day's work a week saved, or the time you can never find to write that novel.

- Drink slowly—put your glass down between sips. Have plenty of water to quench thirst before you start drinking. Alternate an alcoholic drink with a nonalcoholic one. If you like white wine, a spritzer (half soda water, tonic, or sparkling mineral water) will help.

- Buy wine and beer with lower alcohol content. Wines, especially, are much stronger than they once used to be—a percentage alcohol content of 13 to 14 percent is nowadays almost typical.

- If you use alcohol to relax, try other means—walking, yoga, meditation, or listening to music.

- When trying to cut down on alcohol intake, avoid situations that make you want a drink.

mind matters

Most of us suffer from periods of stress, depression, anxiety, or brain overload from time to time, but if they are too frequent or long-lasting, this can truly affect the quality of your life. This chapter explores the solutions that can work for you.

For many people, midlife is a time when a lot of the negative feelings of youth—shyness, lack of confidence, excessive worrying over trifles, for example—have faded and been replaced with more positivity, increased self-worth and the comforting feeling we "know who we are" and know our place in the world.

However, it is still easy for life to run out of control when we least expect it, causing us to have to rethink what makes us happy, what makes us sad—what makes our mind work well or what causes it to show signs of breaking down. For other people, it is that very feeling of being "in a rut," dependable, responsible, or may be even "left behind" that makes us feel miserable. "Going nowhere syndrome" is understandably the cause of much depression.

Stress also isn't the preserve of the young. For some in their 40s and 50s, even if we may be not achieving a lot in terms of personal progress, but are still nurturing others, it can take up a lot of time, effort, and energy to do so, and leave us hanging on like leaves in a storm. Anxiety over the "typical" problems of midlife, such as divorce, severance, or bereavement, can also be hard to cope with. Sometimes there might not be an obvious cause for mental or emotional problems. Then, altering simple lifestyle factors can often change your mood or affect your mental health.

These pages will help you decide whether your mind problems are worthy of concern. Short questionnaires are provided—test yourself to find out if you are suffering from too many of the signs of depression, anxiety, or stress. If so, use the tips on improving your outlook and situation. Finally, we help you to tune up your memory and conserve your brain power, summarizing all the latest advice on retaining mental agility for years to come.

depression is one of the most common complaints of all, suffered by nearly everyone at some point in their lives. One of the most difficult thing is recognizing the signs of depression and admitting to it.

Depression affects 24 percent of women around the menopause, and a quarter of men between the ages of 55 and 65. Being depressed not only feels horrible, but can adversely affect your health—research shows depressed people's immune system is lowered, causing them to get more coughs and colds. Profound periods of depression can even help to cause early death through cancer and cardiovascular disease, researchers at the Danish Epidemiology Science Center have determined.

Although a tendency to depression can be hereditary, it is often "circumstantial," following a bereavement, disappointment, or other negative life event. It can also be hormonal (for example, in women, before a period or during menopause). Other causes of depression have been named as using the computer for more than five hours a day, lack of exercise, boredom, lack of sunlight (season-al affective disorder/SAD), and some illnesses – thyroid disease can cause a depressivelike state, for example.

In chronic depression, the balance of brain chemicals is altered and treatment via prescription drugs (usually SSRIs, see page 176) might be necessary to restore the status quo, but there are several self-help methods to help you overcome it. Getting started is the hardest step, as depression can leave you unwilling to even get out of bed.

Research shows depressed people do best at first with gentle exercise in a noncompetitive environment—swimming or yoga are ideal. Three 30-minute sessions a week of walking lead to a greater boost in mood than SSRIs, one study found.

Comfort eating is a cliché, but some foods and supplements can help to boost feelings of well-being. A generally healthy diet, high in complex carbohydrates (see Chapter 1), insures good brain function, while any serotonin-boosting food (see page 189) will help. Depression can be linked with folate and selenium deficiency—eat plenty of folate-rich foods, such as leafy greens and fortified breakfast cereals, and find selenium in Brazil nuts and variety meat. Avoid drowning your sorrows in alcohol as this can actually lower your mood farther.

Supplements of St.-John's-Wort are mild antidepressants, while 5-HTP and omega-3 fish oils might also work. SAD can be alleviated by means of light therapy (using special lamps or light bulbs)—home-use equipment can be purchased via the Internet or mail order. Essential oils and perfumes can lift mood—citrus, neroli, green tea and rosemary are uplifting. Upbeat music is a great mood-enhancer, especially if you dance—not just listen—and laughter produces body chemicals that enhance mood. Of course, you don't feel like laughing when you are depressed, but ask someone to bring you a comedy video or book and you might find yourself laughing nonetheless.

If depression lasts longer than two weeks, see your doctor.

signs of depression

The more ticks, the more likely it is that you are depressed.

- Loss of interest in the activities you normally enjoy
- Low energy levels
- Poor concentration
- Low self-esteem
- Crying easily
- Inability to make decisions
- Excessive need for sleep OR insomnia
- Feelings of hopelessness
- Low libido
- Suicidal/self-harm thoughts

anxiety is described as "intense apprehension that may or may not have an obvious cause." The most common form—persistent anxiety state—is most likely to begin in midlife, affecting more women than men.

Temporary anxiety is a normal and useful reaction to situations that might be harmful to us, so we are better prepared to deal with them. For example, you feel nervous because you see a bull approaching your footpath, so you move away; you feel anxious because your report is due to be filed in an hour, so you work harder. There is also good research that shows bursts of anxiety can actually boost the immune system. However, frequent bouts for no real reason, or a permanent state of nervousness, can wreck lives.

Some people seem to have a naturally more nervous disposition than others, which is probably genetic. Such people are likely to be slim and energetic, rarely still. That heightened state of anxiety compared with the laid-back, slower neighbor only matters if it matters to you. Persistent anxiety state (PAS) is the term for when you have excessive, frequent or long-term anxiety you can't control, while panic disorder consists of bouts of intense anxiety combined with physical symptoms, which can occur even when there is little to worry about.

Sometimes PAS can include panic disorder. With panic disorder, it is advisable to see your doctor, who might refer you for cognitive behaviour therapy (CBT) and/or medication. Persistent anxiety can also need medical help, and can also benefit from CBT but there are several ways you may be able to help yourself.

Relaxation exercises, such as deep breathing, meditation, stretching, and yoga (see Chapter 2), can calm anxiety. For short-term nerves, such as before a stage performance, high-energy exercise is best—for example, skipping. Massage can relax the mind and reduce anxiety. Calming music or sounds, such as chill-out or waves, work for short-term anxiety. Focusing on situations that worry you and visualizing yourself dealing with them in a positive successful way is useful.

Hypnotherapy with a trained consultant helps some people and is especially helpful if your anxiety is specific and short-term, such as giving a speech, or is phobia-based, such as a fear of spiders. The supplement Relora (extract of magnolia) has been shown in clinical trials to reduce anxiety and stress. Remember short-term worry in itself is fairly harmless—what can do the damage is anxiety about worrying.

signs of anxiety

The more you can tick, the more likely it is that you have a high level of anxiety.

- Sense of foreboding with no obvious reason
- Inability to relax physically
- Brain won't slow down or unwind, particularly at bedtime
- Insomnia
- Inability to concentrate on a book, film, newspaper article
- Worrying thoughts which won't go away
- Abdominal cramps, nausea
- Loose bowels
- Frequent visits to the bathroom to urinate
- Perspiration, hot flashes
- Trembling hands
- Difficulty swallowing
- Shortness of breath or dizziness
- Palpitations

The top 10 things we worry about: Money, personal health, work performance, losing our job and/or retirement, health of family, relationships, getting older, the way we look, not being fit or slim; the world around us.

stress might be defined as unacceptable pressures inflicted on you in the short or long term that result in a wide range of potentially negative physical and emotional reactions.

All of us feel stress at some time, which is normal and can actually be productive and good for us. When we are stressed, hormones, such as adrenaline, are released to increase arousal, energy, strength, and performance, thus helping us get through busy periods or difficult things.

In modern life, though, stress can easily become overwhelming and/or the normal state, and it is then that we may need to find ways to reduce it. Long-term living under constant stress, whether physical or mental, can exacerbate, or is linked with, all the following conditions: high blood pressure due to increased heartbeat, and central fat distribution (big belly) due to extra circulating cortisol, the "stress hormone," both of which increase the risk of cardiovascular disease; digestive disorders, such as ulcers, constipation, and irritable bowel syndrome; insomnia; reliance on alcohol or drugs; impotence; muscular pain; burn-out/nervous breakdown; impaired memory; and a variety of mental disorders. Stress can also affect your immune system and leave you more prone to infection and even cancer.

These effects can be more frequent or more apparent for people in midlife who have been under stress for many years. So if you feel that you are stressed out, it is time to take action to reduce the stress and/or help your body to cope.

coping with stress

A healthy diet will provide all the vitamins and minerals your body needs to help it cope with stress. Particularly important are vitamin C and the B group, which are depleted more quickly under stress and can't be stored in the body.

Supplements of zinc, magnesium, and echinacea help boost the immune system against stress-induced illness; a diet high in antioxidants helps repair the free-radical damage caused by long-term stress, and you can also try Relora (extract of magnolia) to help you through short-term

high-stress periods. For stress that is based on anger, frustration, or any emotion, exercise is vital—short bursts of intense interval training (or even plate-smashing), with plenty of rest in between, are good, but any kind of physical activity will help to disperse adrenaline and cortisol.

Physical contact, such as stroking, massage, or touching, has been shown to produce hormones called oxytocins that reduce stress, especially in women. Short-term stress-relievers include good sex, "palming" your eyes with your hands, yawning, stretching, or a cup of camomile tea.

Get enough sleep (see pages 188–9). Never work more than four hours at one sitting or nine

signs of stress

The more you tick, the more likely you are suffering from stress.

- You work more than forty-five hours a week.
- You easily "fly off the handle" or exhibit grumpiness.
- You are sometimes irrational.
- You have a poor memory.
- You have trouble concentrating.
- You jump out of your skin at a sudden noise.
- You have insomnia.
- You have a lot of fat around your abdomen.
- You feel exhausted much of the time, and no better in the mornings.
- You frequently have an upset stomach.
- You regularly use alcohol and/or drugs.
- You often feel you are about to "crack up."
- You have low libido.
- You sometimes get chest pains but do not have a heart condition.
- Your muscles often ache or hurt and/or you often feel stiff.
- You get dizzy spells.
- You often cancel social engagements or have little time for friends.
- You succumb to a lot of small illnesses and often feel unwell.

Mr Grumpy? It's all in the hormones ● Irritability is a sign of stress—and research (admittedly on sheep!) shows that declining testosterone levels increase irritability. (See Andropause, pages 174 and 177.) ● Scientists have found a gene, 5-HTT, which has two versions, one sensitive, the other coping. Depending on which our DNA has, we can cope well with stress or succumb to it. So don't feel guilty, blame your genes instead!

hours in one day. Learn to say "no" and stop trying to be an all-people pleaser. Plan for 15 minutes' total peace and quiet once every day, or in three 5-minute sessions (excluding sleep time). Maintain a balance between home, work, family, and friends.

Alzheimer's disease

People with poor memory in midlife or younger don't necessarily go on to get Alzheimer's disease, but forgetfulness is the first-stage sign. Alzheimer's is a degenerative brain disease that causes nerve cells to die, so the brain shrinks and its structure and chemical content changes character. It is estimated that by 2050, 14 million Americans will have Alzheimer's, and worldwide the number might reach 45 million.

Very modest drinking of alcohol (up to 1 glass a day) might help prevent dementia, while regular drinking of more than 1 glass actually increases the risk. Poor blood supply to the brain (often caused by atherosclerosis, or hardening of the arteries) is thought to increase the risk, too—regular aerobic exercise, avoidance of smoking, a diet low in saturated fat and high in fish oils, fruit, and vegetables can counteract this, and gingko biloba might also help by keeping the arteries connected to the brain supple and free from clogging. Folate supplements lower the blood concentration of homocysteine—high levels of this amino acid double the risk of Alzheimer's, it has been found.

Aspirin or other antiinflammatory drugs (NSAIDs), taken daily over a long period, lower the risk by 70 percent. HRT for postmenopausal women and THT (testosterone treatment) for men might also lower the risk, although this is yet to be proved. There is also still debate over whether aluminum (in drinking water and/or from aluminum pans) is linked, as Alzheimer's seems to be most common in areas with highest levels of aluminum in the water.

memory

In midlife, many people complain their memory is much worse than it was even a few years before. Powers of memory, mental flexibility, and reasoning are associated with the frontal lobes of the brain, the power of which tends to decline as we age. This decline can be kept at bay with a variety of strategies. (Farther advice on maintaining brain power appears in the next Chapter.)

● Some supplements can help. In tests, Siberian ginseng improved information storage and retrieval; gingko biloba might aid memory by improving blood flow to the brain; soy isoflavones might boost receptors in the hippocampus (the brain's memory area); phosphatidyl serine improves the action of brain neurotransmitters and might slow memory decline.

● Poor memory is a symptom of thyroid disorder—get yourself checked out if you also have tiredness, constipation and/or feel cold all the time.

● Oily fish or fish oil supplements might help boost memory.

● Memory loss can be associated with depression, stress, and anxiety.

● People with a high IQ and/or who have intellectual stimulation and an active social life generally suffer less from memory loss.

● Folate supplements lower blood levels of the amino acid homocysteine—high levels double the risk of Alzheimer's. As with poor memory, keeping the brain active will help stave off Alzheimer's.

5

time for your newlife

Who are you now? The earlier years of midlife are so tremendously busy for most of us that you might—when there is eventually a breathing space—suddenly realize you have no idea who you really are any more, it has been so long since you had the time or energy to think about your own needs.

As our allotted life span gets longer and longer, most of us are hardly more than halfway through our lives when we get to 50 or so. How will you spend the thirty, forty, or fifty years you may have ahead? Do you know what you want to do?

Midlife is an ideal time for making changes and choices, for finding new roles to play, for getting in touch with the present, and making plans for the future. And yet, often none of that happens. All too frequently we settle for cozy familiarity or, worse, resign ourselves to what life is, rather than what it can be.

But we all must change and move on, whether we like it or not. And change is what helps to keep us young and enthusiastic. Chapter 5 helps you to get the most out of your life, and to answer that question—Who are you now?

so you have good health, a good diet, good looks, and a fit body What are you going to do with it all?

While a typical young person tends to grab opportunities as they speed by—and feels that a year in a job is an aeon; that "new" is good and "old" is less good—one of the most common markers of passing youth has often been seen as a growing reluctance to change in ideas, direction, lifestyle, or character; to hang on to what is there; to accept this is "the beginning of the end."

In recent decades, however, we have realized midlife is the end of nothing, but a new start. It is time to "go for it"—whatever "it" might be. Indeed, research shows it is people who embrace innovation gladly and who lead what is always termed a "full and active life" who live longer, and appear younger than their years.

Of course, there are parts of your life you are right not to want to change and would, indeed, be foolish so to do—a happy marriage, for example. And there is nothing wrong with being quiet and contemplative, enjoying your own company, or not wanting to move from the home you've lived in for the past twenty years. These are your strong and stable foundations—recognizing them as such but not being frightened to add new elements is what will always make you feel alive.

Chapter 5 helps you to decide what you really want, and to deal with times in your life when matters are decided for you.

The first section of the chapter, Making It Your Way, is, if you like, the sly kick to make you take that slightly frightening leap of faith, or sometimes the gently encouraging friend —which is often all you need. It is full of ideas and decision-making tools.

Of course, there are a lot of things you can't change—a death in the family, for example, or a job severance. The Letting Go chapter offers advice on dealing with change that is forced upon you, and looks at the difficult period when the children "fly the nest."

Streamline Your Life is where we appraise your time, and how you use it. Midlife can often be more "time-poor" than any other period, so there is help with organizing your days and forward-planning. We also consider how to keep your brain sharp and efficient. Many people have to make a decision about whether to work or retire, whether to commute or work from home—we help you weigh up the options.

Finally, we look at your changing relationship with your family and friends, your elderly relatives, and your social life. Some people say the only real friends you ever make are when you are young ... but, as we shall see, that is simply not true.

It really is time for your new life now—let's get going.

making it your way

If you can't do what you want now, today, this week, this year—when can you do it? Midlife is not only the best, but also the most important time to find yourself, be yourself, please yourself, and enjoy yourself. And that doesn't actually mean you have to change into an extremely selfish person, or feel guilty.

Life at any age is all about balance, but too often during the busy, busy years of the 20s, 30s, and often 40s your own needs, pleasures, and concerns have to take a back seat. You tend to put yourself last. Women, in particular those mixing career with family, are adept at doing this, but it is by no means a female preserve. Many men work long hours for perhaps a large salary but little other reward and still have to play many roles at home—protector, home handyman expert, gardener, chef, whatever—as well.

So, when you reach the late 40s or 50s you need and deserve to recognize your own life is as important as anyone else's. The people you know and love should actually benefit from your recognition of this fact, although they may take a while to realize it!.

Given the modern gift of a period of many years after the age of 50 of reasonable health and comparative wealth and free time, it really IS time to be your own person. So in this section we look at all the ways you might make some changes and choices that will, hopefully, have you feeling more content, more alive and happier than you have been for some time. In midlife many people make changes only when forced to by a "wake-up call," but often when this happens we find we wish we had made those changes a long time ago.

First, do the questionnaire overleaf to find out how much of a rut you are in, then use the idea on the following pages to help you decide how things might improve. From enjoying your new place in the 'pecking order," to seeking anything from tranquillity to excitement, there is plenty of choice.

All it takes is some self-belief and confidence to dig out what you really want and work out how to get it. Go on—why NOT cram in a few detours, adventures, and challenges, rather than later having to ponder on what might have been?

are you in a rut?

Answer the following 10 questions honestly, choosing the answer that most nearly matches your experience if there isn't one that is exactly right, then calculate whether you have ticked more As, more Bs, or more Cs, and check your profile below.

1 how long is it since you cooked a new recipe?
a) 1 week or less
b) 1 to 3 months
c) About a year

2 how often do you buy yourself something new to wear?
a) Every month or less
b) Twice a year
c) Hardly ever

3 how often do you look at a daily newspaper different from your regular one?
a) Once a week or less
b) Now and then
c) Never

4 when did you last have a weekend away from home not related to work?
a) Within the past 2 months
b) Within the past 6 months
c) Rarely have weekends away

5 when choosing your major annual vacation, which of these options do you go for?
a) Go to a new country every year
b) Go to the same area, but in different accommodation
c) Always go to the same resort and same accommodation

6 TV—do you have the following?
a) Satellite TV with all the stations
b) Satellite, but only the basic free channels
c) Only terrestrial channels

7 how long is it since you made friends with anyone new?
a) This past year
b) 2 to 3 years
c) More than 5 years

8 when did you last voluntarily do something that made you feel a bit nervous, afraid, or unsure?
a) Within the past 2 months
b) Within past year
c) Can't remember

9 how long is it since you learned a new skill, such as a hobby or language, not related to work?
a) Within the past year
b) Within the past 5 years
c) Can't remember

10 what is your view of the Internet?
a) Great—use it all the time
b) We have a computer, but I don't really know what I am doing
c) Don't like the idea; don't have a computer

scoring

Mostly As: You are most certainly not in a rut—don't lose your sense of adventure as you get older, it is what keeps people feeling young and living longer. A 2002 survey found that it is boredom, more than stress or lack of money, that diminishes a sense of well-being as we age.

Mostly Bs: That rut is looking dangerously close and you have one foot in it. You're in danger of stagnating, so it is time to reinvent areas of your life and see what adventures are out there for the taking.

Mostly Cs: Oh dear! You fell into a rut a while ago and you can't seem to get yourself out—perhaps you don't even think you want to. But you need to get up and dust yourself off. As they say— this is no rehearsal, this is your life.

So, did my little questionnaire show that you ARE in a rut, or borderline? It is surprising how infrequently many of us even bother to think about what we do each day as we get older. We just get up and get on with today much as we did yesterday. If nothing awful happens, then it is a good day.

There is, however, more to your life than that. Sometimes you need to be brave and bold to change things, that's all. You have that capacity. Indeed, new research shows that, while in the past people over the age of 41 rarely made voluntary major changes to their lives, now we are actually more willing to change jobs, households, partners, or lifestyles than ever before.

You might feel you don't have the time … that life is far too busy to worry about making changes that can cost effort and stress you out even more. So, if time is your problem, go to pages 222–7 for help. If you do have time, however, start thinking and planning now about how you would like your life to be. You need to make this time and make sure you are focused on your thoughts. Take a walk on your own to begin with, or sit alone in a quiet room in a comfortable chair. If you are going to write your ideas down, use a pen and some paper, not the computer. Try to build yourself some mental pictures as you take these 3 steps.

redefine your base
See what you already have and take a fresh new look at it. Family. Work. Home. How are you coping with changes in the pecking order? Once your children grow up you have a different role to play (see Family and Friendships, pages 228–35). Accept that things change and you need to change with them (for more on this, see Letting Go, pages 216–21).

Make a list of all the things in your life make you happy, that you don't want to change. This defines what you have achieved in life so far and gives you a good springboard. Try to recall when you were a child—the wonder and joy you felt at quite ordinary things, sometimes just at the simple fact of being alive. And think about the importance of keeping an open mind to opinions and possibilities.

find the right balance
This is such a terrific time to get balance back into your life after what has probably been a mad few years. Apart from health, balance is probably the most important factor in living a happy and long life. Think back to when you were a young adult. What were your hopes, dreams, and ambitions then? How many got forgotten or pushed aside? We all have wishes we have never fulfilled; some will no longer be what we want at all, while some can be still be achieved.

Ask yourself some questions about how much of the following you have in your life:
⬤ Peace? ⬤ Excitement? ⬤ Innovation? ⬤ Friends? ⬤ A close family? ⬤ Culture? ⬤ Information? ⬤ Beauty? ⬤ Challenge? ⬤ Spirituality? ⬤ Work? ⬤ Leisure?

See if you can pinpoint areas where you can get more; areas that are too much. Think about how you can create or restore balance.

make plans
Now it is time to make lists and plans. The discussion overleaf on retirement might help you decide on the right work/leisure balance for you. The ideas on pages 214–15 might give you some inspiration for different things to do with your time.

Write your own list of things you want to do. Divide the list into three—Big Things (start your own business from home; write that best-selling novel), Little or Medium Things (call some old friends, decorate the kitchen), and Self-Improvement Things (learn a new language, try to stop being so negative). Discuss the list with your partner, if you have one.

Finally, make a plan of how, when, and where you are going to do these things. I would suggest making this plan realistic. If you have brought up a family or run any kind of business, you will know how to make schedules that can be kept to.

Pick a few "big," "little," and "self-improvement" things to do in the next year. Look at the plan—is there a good mix? Pin it up somewhere. Start on one thing from each of the three sections immediately. Don't rely on things happening without you making them happen. Research shows that people create their own luck . Those who think of themselves as "lucky" tend to be optimists who exploit opportunities and listen to their own intuition.

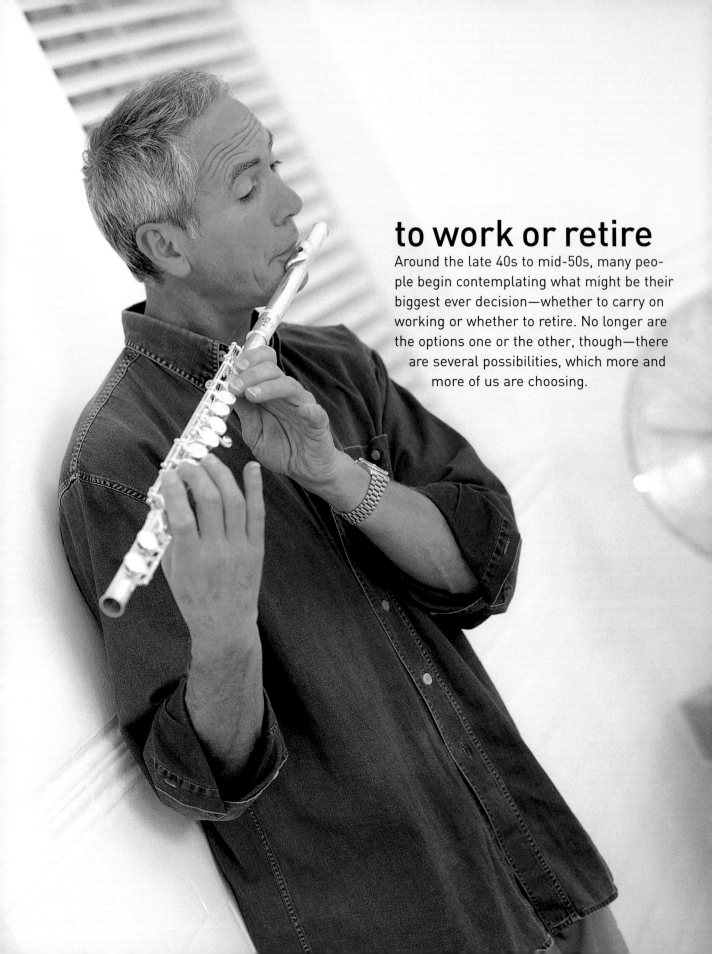

to work or retire

Around the late 40s to mid-50s, many people begin contemplating what might be their biggest ever decision—whether to carry on working or whether to retire. No longer are the options one or the other, though—there are several possibilities, which more and more of us are choosing.

full retirement This is no longer always unavoidable at 60 or 65, as it was for so long for so many of us. In most careers, whether high-flying or undemanding, you no longer have to be "pensioned off" (what a horrible term!) at a certain age if you don't want to be. Many people choose to carry on working, not just because of the extra money, but because they enjoy work and/or are worried that there won't be much in life for them if they do retire.

However, when—inevitably—retirement is impending, for many people it really does seem to spell "the end," with little left to look forward to except physical decline. If you dread the thought of retiring, first banish the "R" word from your vocabulary. Instead think of yourself as being allowed to start afresh. Try not to be afraid, try not to avoid thinking about the moment, and do what those who are happy to retire do—plan ahead. Open your mind to possibilities, start making lists as early as possible beforehand and don't discount anything or anyone who can enrich your "retirement" years. See the panel on the right for ideas on other work you can do.

If you don't want to—or are not able to—carry on working and yet still don't feel happy to retire, it might be because you feel your home life or partner relationship is poor or unfulfilling. In that case, read Family and Friendships, pages 228–35.

severance This can be worse mentally than normal-age retirement, even if cushioned with a payoff. Check out the panel on the right for ideas on how to get back into work mode.

choosing to retire One survey of working women found that their main causes of stress were work-related: 51 percent cited heavy workload, 42 percent lack of leisure time, 34 percent trouble-making work colleagues and 21 percent bad bosses/ employees. No wonder many women

new ways of working

If you don't want to carry on in your old job in the same way, but you don't really want to go for full retirement, weigh up some of these options:

- **work part-time** or job share.
- **see if you can do your job from home** either full time or at least on certain days of the week.
- **take a year off,** then return to your old job— more and more 40+ people are doing this. One way to fund it is to rent out your home for the year.
- **try seasonal** or voluntary work.
- **apply for a new job** Many people find new employment whatever their age. A survey reveals 50 percent of retired people who later decide to go to return to work get a job without any problem.
- **retrain** The largest percentage of students returning to education in adulthood are women over 40.
- **start your own business** If you have no mortgage now, or have severance money or savings, or can find a sponsor, it might be time to start a small business, whether in a similar area to your old career or on a completely new tack. Either way, it will pay you to plan ahead and not leave your old job until you have everything in place as far as possible. At least make sure you have done your research/found your gap in the market and know how you plan to make things work.
- **work from home** With communications now being so good, you can move to the country/seaside/abroad and still do a wide variety of work from home.
- **use your home** A large house can be a guest house or country hotel; a large garden might be a herb garden center or a boarding kennels. Great cook? You can make produce to sell. Ex-photographer/designer/captain of industry? You can run weekend courses in your specialist field.

a recent survey found that the top five factors that effect well-being are: ● Feeling in control ● Having an optimistic outlook ● Being content with your appearance ● Having a sense of belonging in the community ● Having good relationships with family and friends. **Work didn't come into the equation at all!**

can't wait to retire once they are over 50! No doubt similar questioning of men—who often get work-related depression in midlife, when they may be passed over for promotion, or can be made to feel "past it" performancewise—would reveal similar results.

Research shows that those who have a happy retirement tend to have a family or partner rather than living on their own, and have a circle of friends (not all work comrades) and outside interests, hobbies, and so on.

One of the main keys to a successful retirement seems to be – long before the actual retirement date – thinking about what you will do with your lovely new free time. Surprisingly, having a lot of money isn't one of the most important factors. A study of 300 people between the ages of 55 and 75 found good health and a small network of close friends were far more important than wealth in retirement. Two other studies in recent years have found similar results. It is only if annual income per head drops below one-third of the average that being poor brings unhappiness, according to one of the reports.

Of course, if all your "wish list" retirement items rely on money for fulfilment, but you are not as wealthy as you would like, then you may have a problem until you contemplate the saying, "Money can't buy you happiness. It only helps you look for it in a lot more places."

choosing to carry on working

Research has found that people who work past their "official" retiring age are, not surprisingly, wealthier than people who take early or normal-age retirement. The same study also found that they tend to be healthier—three-quarters of working men aged 55 to 75 described their health as excellent or very good, compared with only 50 percent of those who had retired.

However, another London-based study of 800 men found the mental functioning of the retired men was better.

In 2002, one study estimated 2.5 million men and 1.9 million women, aged over 65, were working or actively seeking employment. It is estimated that about one-third of all retirees are doing paid work. More and more employers are realizing early retirement is a waste of talent, experience, skill, and expertise. Perhaps the best option for people who would like to continue working over 65, but who need more leisure-related balance in their lives, is to check out other "halfway" options—see page 213.

boredom or burn out While you

might not want to give up work, you might be feeling almost terminally bored with your actual job, or you might be suffering from burnout. More and more people in their 40s and 50s are changing career, changing tack, or finding other ways out of the work rut. If you feel trapped at work for any reason, it is always best to find an exit strategy. We all need change to stir ourselves up. If you leave a job you no longer enjoy, you have lost nothing except your income. Although this can be more than scary, downsizing early can be rewarding and life-enhancing. Also see page 213 for income-generating ideas.

do something different...

10

ways to spice up your life

The Internet has details of many of the ideas mentioned here. Note that people in poor health or with a physical disability are not advised to try some of the more demanding suggestions.

1 Read your way through the Top 100 all-time favorite books. Be sure you have an up-to-date library card.

2 Take to the skies—depending on your fear-factor level, go hot-air-ballooning/gliding/microlighting/sky diving.

3 Do someone else a favor—whether it's a sponsored charity walk or shopping for a sick neighbor, helping others, research shows, makes us more cheerful.

4 Book up a course of sessions with a life coach.

5 Go for a weekend camping in a tent—everyone should do it once in their lives.

6 Set yourself a physical challenge—climb Kilimanjaro, run a half-marathon, walk the Appalachin Trail, learn gymnastics, or salsa dancing.

7 Have a spa weekend on your own, with all the treatments and a light diet.

8 Plan a home-swap vacation (you go to someone's home for your vacation and they come to yours)—it's less expensive and more fun than a hotel or apartment vacation.

9 Go to a amusement park and take one of the scary rides—or at least, go on the old-fashioned merry-go-round with the dancing horses and eat some popcorn or candy floss.

10 Go to your local bus station and get on the first bus that comes along (excluding local commuter buses). Go as far as you can in a day and spend the night in a hotel before returning home.

now think of 10 ideas of your own!

letting go

In midlife, most people face an often surprising degree of change—and not always of their own making. Learning to let go and move on is never easy, but unexpected or unwanted changes can be made less traumatic ...

Midlife is when the roots that most of us put down in early adulthood become deep and firm. Years pass by and it can be easy to get lulled into feeling that what you have—how your life is—will stay that way for ever. Often in midlife, though, a long period of equilibrium will be swiftly followed by sudden or unexpected or unwanted change. Sometimes you may see it coming, or, indeed, know it is coming, but at other times it can be a shock.

The most common of these changes are the end of a long-term marriage or relationship, children leaving home or going to university, a parent, partner, or other close person dying, a job severance or forced early retirement, and having to move home or city

All these changes can be—and must be—coped with, but it is rarely easy. Some of us will find it harder to deal with than others. You have to learn to prepare yourself for change, and then to let go after it has happened, and move on. It may even be possible to enjoy change even though you have to face something you always thought you would dread. A change of perspective is often all you really need to wind up realizing that your life can actually improve.

This section discusses each of the most usual "change" situations and how you might cope effectively.

we all have to deal with change

Some people thrive on it—even seek it out—while others fear it and attempt to avoid it. These pages offer guidance on all the major "forced" changes you are likely to meet in midlife and suggests how you might cope with them.

a death in the family

In midlife most people face the death of a loved one—parent, partner, friend—perhaps for the first time, and with it the truth of our own mortality, the inevitability of losing people we love, and of the irreversible nature of death. Once people are gone, you can't tell them you care about them any more, and you can't say sorry. So grief is often colored with guilt and both are hard to bear. If it is a parent who dies, you feel that sense of being orphaned just as if you were ten years old. Now it is up to you to be the "older generation" and—as my husband said after his mother died, "Well, it is our turn next." And the death of a younger person—someone your own age or younger—can be an even greater shock, proving that you are not immortal.

So there is nothing positive to be gained from the experience of death. Well, perhaps there is, although it may not be apparent for some long time. People who have suffered loss often say the death makes them reassess their own lives. It can make you behave differently toward people you care about, can help you to live your life to the full and in the present, rather than thinking about what might have been or procrastinating.

Death can also bring you back in touch with people who were once important to you and/or make you realize how many people do care about you. Indeed, when coping with the death of a partner or other close family member, it is this support that gets most of us through. There are not any shortcuts to coming to terms with the changes a death will bring to you—but letting people into your life, and not putting on a "brave front," are the two ways to begin.

Joining a group of people who are in the same situation as you, or have recently been through it and have survived, has been shown to shorten the period of depression that follows any bereavement. The support, encouragement, and advice you will receive from such a group are invaluable.

moving home

There are two main reasons why you may need to move home now. The first is that you want, or need, to downsize for reasons of finance or convenience. This often accompanies a divorce or split, or a job loss or retirement—so it can often be a double dose of misery for people who don't like change.

If finance is the reason, you need to act quickly before debts mount—and the business of selling, finding somewhere to go, and organizing everything is often a good therapy once you begin. So don't dither—grab the change and take charge. The main decision that needs careful thought is whether to stay in the same area or move away.

The worst part of moving somewhere smaller can be having to divest yourself of treasured possessions and furniture. See if you can offload these on to children, siblings, or other relatives who will appreciate your things (obviously with divorce your ex will take the surplus); otherwise choose carefully what goes and what stays and recognize a good clear-out is symbolic of what is happening in your life. You will almost certainly surprise yourself and find this makes you feel better. If it turns out the old prints in the attic make a lot of money at a yard sale, so much the better—time for a vacation.

You might also decide you need to move for other reasons—to get a new job or be near children or elderly parents, for example. In such cases, the move is at least partly your decision, which does make it easier. So let the decision be right. You need to make a list of pros and cons of the potential move before going ahead, take all the advice you can get, and make sure everyone involved in the decision is consulted.

Once the move is done, you need to strike a balance between keeping in touch with old friends and family and making a new life. For more tips on this, see the discussion on the End of a marriage/relationship (page 220) and the section on Family and Friendships (pages 228–35).

career change/end

When you lose your job, for whatever reason—or perhaps are made bankrupt—there is little more confidence-damaging, as work still fundamentally defines who we are. So why is it that while some collapse in the face of what they see as disaster, perhaps becoming chronically depressed and unable to function, others cope well and finally emerge happier than ever before?

dealing with the fear of change

- Understand that life is dynamic not static, and so are people's needs. If unwanted change happens to you, it isn't necessarily anything you are doing or did wrong. Knowing you are not at fault helps.

- Don't try to preempt change by not living a full life or by clinging to what you have. It won't work and it will make you feel more isolated and worse when change does happen. Take risks and make choices yourself, otherwise others will do it for you.

- Change can seem worse if you feel you have no element of control. For changes that you know will happen eventually – for example, children leaving home – get involved in the build-up to the change rather than ignoring it. For instance, helping children sort out their new lives before they leave will make you feel part of the process and not a helpless bystander.

- Visualize yourself in different situations, such as in a different house, without a job (if you currently have one), or living alone (if you are currently with a partner). Plan what you might do in each of these situations. Always have time each day to visualize what your life can be like. This powerful tool will help you cope if your thoughts become reality.

- For sudden change that can leave you feeling bereft or depressed, remember you can always have professional counseling. Knowing you have this option if anything "bad" happens to you can be a great comfort blanket.

One important factor is having family/partner who don't/doesn't make you feel that their happiness—or your esteem—is dependent upon your income. You also need your own sense of self-worth beyond that provided by your capacity to work and/or earn well. Developing this sense early in adulthood is protection against the depression of "failure" at work. However, it is not too late to nurture it even after the event: see pages 212–14, where we discuss work and retirement. One thing is certain—it isn't too late to seek other employment, and there is little element of luck involved. Research shows that all of us can "get lucky" if we keep optimistic and try hard enough.

end of a marriage/relationship

If your partner wants to leave you—or walks out, or even if they have an affair—research shows this is an even bigger blow to most people than losing a long-term job or business, and almost as bad as if they had died. As some studies estimate that 50 percent of first marriages end in divorce, however, so it is something many of us will have to deal with—especially men, as three-quarters of proceedings are initiated by women.

There are steps you can take to make sure your own long-term relationship doesn't end in a split (see Family and Friendships, pages 228–35). These days an affair needn't be the end of a relationship, and can even make it better (usually with the help of counseling, though). But sometimes you have to admit it just isn't going to work out, and let go. Give yourself a month for every year you were together to come to terms with the change. Of course, this is an average—you can help yourself by making sure you do all you can to insure a "good divorce." It might be possible to split and, eventually (or even sooner), be friends.

If there are offspring, you will feel much better if you can pull off a nonacrimonious divorce. And you can help yourself avoid the loneliness that splitting often brings by keeping in touch with family and friends throughout your marriage/partnership, and by always remembering to have a life that doesn't depend on your partner for its fun or satisfaction.

The needier and more dependent you were in the partnership, the more likely it is you will have to be taught to be happy again—counseling, friends, and family can all help you to do this and it is vital to accept help rather than pushing people away. The two most important things to learn are: if your partner is now your ex, they were a part of your life which was right for then, but not now; and although you are no longer together, what you had and shared is still important and always will be.

children leaving home

When you are a parent with children still living at home, the question, "What shall I do today?" is rarely needed. Over a period of about twenty years, time is automatically filled with seeing to their many needs. Occasional fleeting moments of wondering what happened to the selfish life you used to lead may flicker in your brain, but that is all.

Hence, when suddenly it's all over and the last child leaves you with "empty-nest syndrome," getting back your own life can be a tremendous shock. Then there is the awesome quiet in the house. The lack of loud music, phones ringing, teenagers laughing, shouting. Why is it that all the things you craved—the time to yourself, the peace, the return to civilization as you used to know it—no longer seem quite so appealing?

Don't worry—it might take weeks, or even months, but soon you will remember what it is you were planning to do and why you sometimes craved your own space and time. Hasten this along by not spending your days and evenings sitting by the phone waiting for offspring to ring. By not constantly phoning them yourself (learn to text them instead). By not always being available 24/7 to sort out laundry and love problems.

Fill the house with your own preferred noise, laughter, and shouting by all means, but relish the peace and some selfish time. Most of us have long, long lists of things we want to do—so plan them and do them. You will always be there for your children, but the last thing they need when they leave home is to feel worried about you or, worse, guilty about you. The sooner you fill the gaps they left the better you will feel. And when they do come home or, even better, invite you around to their place, you'll all love each other all the more.

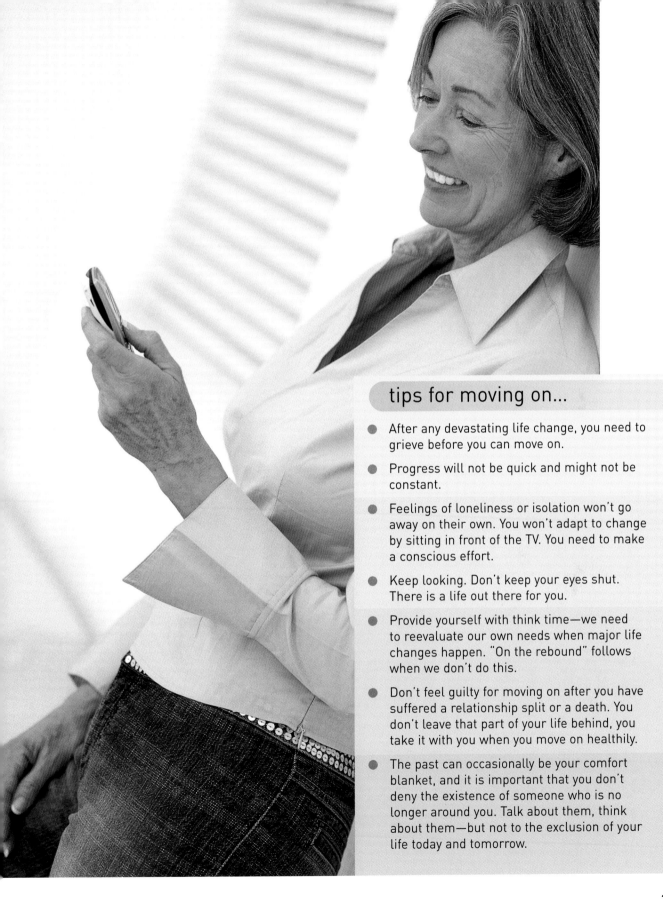

tips for moving on...

- After any devastating life change, you need to grieve before you can move on.

- Progress will not be quick and might not be constant.

- Feelings of loneliness or isolation won't go away on their own. You won't adapt to change by sitting in front of the TV. You need to make a conscious effort.

- Keep looking. Don't keep your eyes shut. There is a life out there for you.

- Provide yourself with think time—we need to reevaluate our own needs when major life changes happen. "On the rebound" follows when we don't do this.

- Don't feel guilty for moving on after you have suffered a relationship split or a death. You don't leave that part of your life behind, you take it with you when you move on healthily.

- The past can occasionally be your comfort blanket, and it is important that you don't deny the existence of someone who is no longer around you. Talk about them, think about them—but not to the exclusion of your life today and tomorrow.

streamline your life

If you never have time to catch your breath, can't decide what to do first on your long list of chores, and rarely get a chance to even think—you need to streamline your life. It's easier than you might imagine.

While the later years of middle age can be relaxed and with plenty of "me" time to spare, those in their 40s and early-to-mid 50s are more likely never to feel their feet touch the floor as they race through life, always seemingly one pace behind where they really need to be.

These years can be more time-poor than any other period. It is also true that the older we get the more quickly days, months, and years seem to go by. This is because when you are, say, five years old, a year represents one-fifth of your whole life to date, and so seems a very long time. When you are 50, a year is only one-fiftieth of your whole life to date and so seems correspondingly shorter.

If you manage to find time to read Streamline Your Life it should help you save a great deal of time. If you often feel your life is surrounded by chaos and muddle, you need it more than most.

We look at how to make each minute count by organizing your days, starting with the most important part of all—planning. This will improve your efficiency. We help you to redefine your priorities—weeding out the unnecessaries from your life and learning how to deal diplomatically with the time-wasting elements and/or people. We see how you can gain extra time by using a few sensible, but often overlooked, strategies. Finally, we look at how to be body-fit and brain-fit for "extra time."

Live by the Rules for Successful Time Management and ... look ... you can suddenly relax!

getting organized
Yes, it does sound boring, but if you want more time for your own needs you just have to get yourself organized. Think of it as freeing yourself up to be able to lead a better, more selfish (in the right sense), and more exciting life.

the importance of planning

First you need to plan ahead—for some reason, women are often better at this than men, but once men get the drift they can make excellent planners. Planning life just as you might make plans in your business is vital, for without it you just wake up in the morning and muddle your way through the day; or you start the week and muddle your way through that, too. So if you are a person who feels time spent thinking is time wasted, then DO think again. Sort your life out logically and you will no longer have to rush around.

Let's find an example. You need food for lunch, so you go to the store and buy ingredients to make soup. Later on, you need food for supper, but you didn't get enough in the morning, so you have to go out again. Next day it is lunchtime and you have nothing to eat, but if you had cooked twice the amount of soup you would not have had to bother about lunch today. Extreme? No—when I'm away from home that is how my husband (dis)organizes his life all the time. But he has plenty of time to fill... Planning ahead could save him or you time both traveling, shopping, and cooking.

how to plan
Make schedules for work and for home life. For both, have a short-term and long-term list of things you have to do. Write the long-term list up once every few weeks in order of importance and tick items off when done. Write the short-term list every couple of days and similarly try to put the hardest or most important tasks first. Psychologically, this helps you to get them done.

Also, think about the order from a practical point of view. Do the chores meld into each other well and save you having to keep chopping and changing modes between them? Never make a journey (even a trip up the stairs at home) without seeing if it can't be used for more than one thing. Example: You go upstairs to find a different pair of shoes to wear. Take up the clean laundry as you go.

Never shop for the short term—buy as much as is practical every trip. Also have a "fun" schedule. Decide on times during the day when you will have a relaxing break, or do some small selfish thing for yourself. If you don't schedule these in it is unlikely that you will do them.

prioritize

The next thing busy people are sometimes poor at is prioritizing. Here's another example. You've been working very long hours for weeks and weeks, seven days a week, to get a project done. You are exhausted and have had no social life at all. The phone rings. It is a teacher from your child's old school, asking if you will go and give a half-day talk to some pupils about a topic that you specialize in. What do you say? Well, you say "yes," of course. Extreme? No—I did it myself not long ago. Why? Because it IS hard to say no. But sometimes you have to.

how to prioritize
Spend a while with computer or paper and pen, prioritizing.

First your obligations. Make a list of things which are nonnegotiable. These might be a certain number of hours at work, commuting, sleeping, showering, etc. Then a list of the things you have to do, but which you can spend less time on and get away with it. These might be, at home, cooking or housework, or, at work, checking e-mails or reading reports. In fact, if you work, make a separate list of how you might save time in the workplace. Unless you are tied to set hours, this will cut down the time you spend there. If you do have set hours, at least you will be less stressed out at work with fewer chores to do.

10 rules for successful time management

- Recognize the areas in which you are not being time-efficient.

- Prioritize using your own values, not someone else's.

- Never allow your time to be totally engulfed with work and obligations. Always factor in time for family, friends, leisure, health, and so on.

- Do harder or less welcome tasks early in the day—not only is your brain usually better able to cope at this time, but it also helps you to feel better about yourself, and therefore more efficient, for the remainder of the day.

- At the end of the day, know what you intend to do tomorrow. At the end of the week, know what you intend to do next week. This helps you to relax and unwind overnight/over the weekend. Even if things don't exactly go according to plan, at least you have a base from which to work.

- Don't aim for perfection. Aim to do as good a job on each task as you can reasonably expect in the time.

- When doing a task, focus 100 percent on it. It will get done quicker and better.

- Don't let pleasures become pressures too. When you feel that trip to the squash court or the drama club is too much like work, give it a rest.

- Always factor in "chill" time every day. Sometimes you need to just do nothing.

- Take help when it is offered—and if it isn't offered, ask for it.

Cheer up—you DO have more time! Life is getting longer. The average American is now expected to live for 77.6 years, with women living for 80.1 years and men 74.8 years. Positive thinking can also add years to your life—on average someone with a cheerful and positive outlook lives 7.5 years longer than a gloomy person.

Now a list of things you can get someone else to do. Delegate or pay someone else to do things, especially those that you are not so good at, or don't enjoy.

Then a list of things you do out of habit, but which might be a waste of your time. These might include watching TV every night (even the programs you don't enjoy); reading trash magazines that other people bring home; surfing the Internet aimlessly; or lying in bed too long at the weekend. Decide what you could cut back on without loss of pleasure in life.

Lastly, make a list of things you do that you really don't want to do and which aren't necessary. This might include the talk at the school, chairing a local committee, keeping in touch with a friend you haven't really got on well with for years, and so on.

Now go through your lists and work out how much time you can save just on having the right priorities in life. You can now use some of the time you save on what you really want to do.

ways to make more time

Here we look at all the other factors apart from prioritizing and planning that can affect your ability to make the most of your time. You need energy. When you are feeling refreshed and full of energy you can skate through twice as much work/housework/reading etc. as when you are lethargic physically or mentally (it's hard to separate the two).

If you are physically fit—with both strength and stamina—you can, obviously, do physical work more quickly. Jobs like housework, gardening, and shopping will all be easier. If your body is fit, your circulation will be in optimum shape, which, in turn, will mean that your brain works well (see opposite). Read Exercise for Energy (pages 86–9).

Watch your stress levels—although in the short-term stress can be a good thing and you might seem to have much more energy than usual because of the extra adrenaline it releases, if you are under constant stress in the long term your energy will suffer. (For more on stress, see pages 202–3.)

you need to think laterally You're
energetic and organized—but you still don't seem to have enough time in the day. Try some of these ideas:

Pay! Recognize you are not always the best person to do a task and don't feel guilty for employing help if you are time-poor. Never feel guilty for employing cleaners, window cleaners, child carers, and so on. Even use a lifestyle manager if necessary (someone who will buy kid's clothes, presents, keep the household organized—in fact, do everything the old-fashioned "wife and mother"—or, these days, "househusband and father"—might have done.)

If you do have to provide meals either for yourself or a houseful, always buy prepared vegetables, salads, cuts of meat, etc. Buy deli goods rather than the more mass-market meals and ingredients. Buy luxury (oysters, caviar) or honest top-quality healthy foods (stone-baked breads, perfect olive oil) if you are time-poor. Complicated recipes can only be for people who don't buy the best!

Get multitasking You can talk, listen, write, and think at the same time when you get used to it, especially if you are brain-fit (see opposite) and well rested. (See Insomnia and sleep, pages 188–9.)

Use white lies. It is easy to get a boring person, who is repeating themselves for the fifth time, off the telephone if you say you have to go because someone is at the door/has arrived for a meeting/you have to rush off etc. etc. In emergencies, disconnect your voice-mail and e-mail, which will save lots of time replying to messages left.

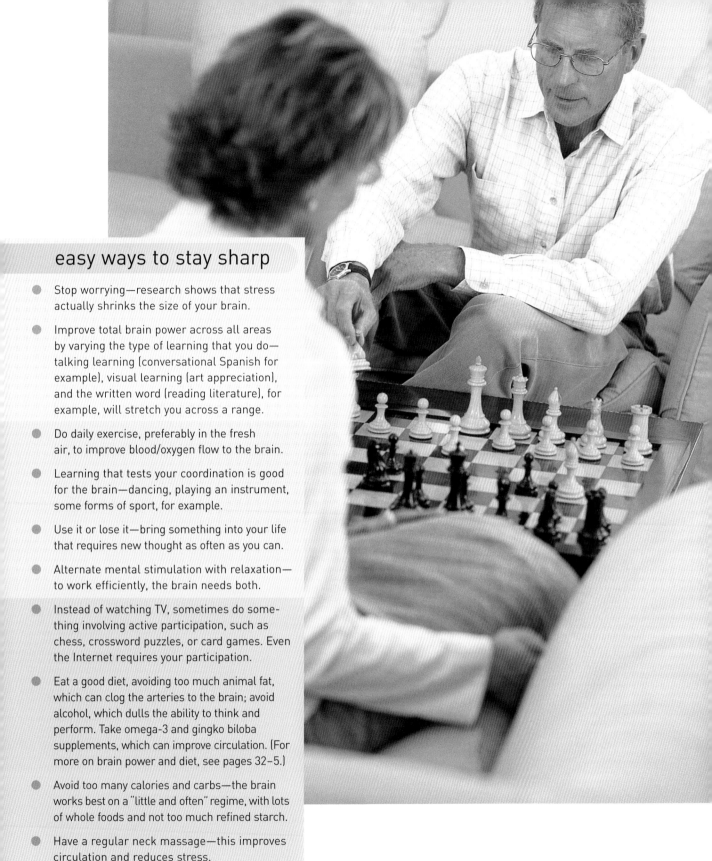

easy ways to stay sharp

- Stop worrying—research shows that stress actually shrinks the size of your brain.

- Improve total brain power across all areas by varying the type of learning that you do—talking learning (conversational Spanish for example), visual learning (art appreciation), and the written word (reading literature), for example, will stretch you across a range.

- Do daily exercise, preferably in the fresh air, to improve blood/oxygen flow to the brain.

- Learning that tests your coordination is good for the brain—dancing, playing an instrument, some forms of sport, for example.

- Use it or lose it—bring something into your life that requires new thought as often as you can.

- Alternate mental stimulation with relaxation—to work efficiently, the brain needs both.

- Instead of watching TV, sometimes do something involving active participation, such as chess, crossword puzzles, or card games. Even the Internet requires your participation.

- Eat a good diet, avoiding too much animal fat, which can clog the arteries to the brain; avoid alcohol, which dulls the ability to think and perform. Take omega-3 and gingko biloba supplements, which can improve circulation. (For more on brain power and diet, see pages 32–5.)

- Avoid too many calories and carbs—the brain works best on a "little and often" regime, with lots of whole foods and not too much refined starch.

- Have a regular neck massage—this improves circulation and reduces stress.

family and friendships

We are all guilty of neglecting our family and friends at least some of the time—and yet what they give us can be more enduring and fulfilling than any career; more comforting than any counselor. Our relationships affect our happiness more than our bank balance does—and that's official, as confirmed by much respected economic and social research. Do you need to do some repair work?

The most important relationship most of us are likely to have is a marriage or other similar long-term commitment to another person. Indeed, plenty of research shows that people who are married tend to be happier and healthier than people who live alone. Surprising, then, that marriage is on the decrease, divorce is now commonplace, and a large percentage of people over the age of 50 live on their own.

In this time-deficient twenty-first century world of rush, hustle, stress, and travel, the state of friendship is also suffering. Long-term friendships are rarer than they were fifty years ago, with only a small minority of us still in touch with people we knew before the age of 20. We have acquaintances rather than deep friendships and people sometimes seem as disposable as a tissue.

And when we do know people well and/or in the long term, we tend to abuse those friendships, letting them slide, letting them fade, and finally disappear. And perhaps we treat our life partners worst of all—having affairs, telling lies, taking them for granted… We have all done at least one of those three things.

Yet, it is established that human beings are tribal creatures, we survive best with close and regular contact with others… relationships, friendships, physical contact, emotional closeness. Whether it is with partners, children, siblings, parents, or friends—we cope better if people who know us are a permanent part of our lives.

In this final section we look at the complicated state of modern family relationships and friendships and see what sense we can make of it all.

partnerships Marriage—or long-term living together—is something that, for those of us who have it, we either tend to take for granted, accepting grudgingly that it is OK, or kind of quietly wriggle and niggle and wonder what the hell we are doing with THIS person all this time. We wonder what are we missing.

No wonder so many marriages go awry in the middle years. The so-called midlife crisis sees men and women disappearing off with younger partners, vanishing to go backpacking around the world, or simply to live alone and take up yoga and self-improvement courses. Most splits in partnerships aren't the result of one half of the partnership being wicked or cruel or robbing a bank, or even because of never-ending, full-decibel rows or mental cruelty. Mostly the marriage just runs out of steam, with neither party bothering to invest enough effort to keep it going. Until finally the "grass-might-be-greener" philosophy provides the push.

the four stages of marriage

Psychologists describe four stages to the typical marriage. First, the romantic, lustful stage that lasts from one to three years. Next, the power struggle stage, when you both find your place in the marital pecking order and have bouts of thinking, "What did I ever see in this person?" This lasts for five to ten years. Toward the end of this stage you either split up, compromise, or, occasionally, find that you both want the same things out of life and each other and are "happily married."

The third stage, which comes along gradually, is the "completely-taking-each-other-for-granted" stage, when your sex life often virtually comes to a halt and the partner is part of the furniture, and you accept—but sometimes despise—that person, warts and all. Or occasionally you simply put up with him or her until the kids have left home and you can be off. This stage is obviously vulnerable to either partner having affairs to reaffirm their attractiveness and as an outlet for sex. Stage three can last up twenty years or more, but in a positive marriage can be much shorter or non-existent.

Lastly, should you by any chance get through all that, and learn the lesson that perhaps your partner is quite nice after all—and that there isn't all that much time left to argue—you have the "reward" stage: two people living their peaceful—or sometimes even exciting—years together as friends, partners and lovers in the true sense, sometimes still with a hint of sex there, but if not it doesn't matter. All is well in the world. Sadly only half of all couples reach that stage—or they continue living in Stage Three, until one dies or bails out.

Assuming you have got through stages one and two and are still married but feel things could be better—what can you do to keep the partnership going? First, ask yourself whether you have a basic foundation to the marriage so it is worth working on. When the children have left home is often a good time to do this. If there are grounds for serious complaints on each side—you feel trapped, perhaps, in a marriage that is enslaving, restricting, or oppressive, for example—these need to be worked out before you can begin improvements.

Sometimes this will need the help of a relationship counselor, because, if you haven't talked together for years, it is really hard to begin what can often be awkward conversations, bringing up things that have remained unsaid for years, on your own. Next, should there be any causes for forgiveness, these need to be addressed. Affairs and major fall-outs should be put behind you and forgiven if not completely forgotten.

If your sex life is not what you both want, then see the section on Libido or, again, seek counseling. Should you both have been taking each other for granted, in one way that isn't such a bad thing, but you need to begin valuing your partner again. Writing a list of their good points is a good start.

Their faults? If there are any you still find hard to accept after all this time, perhaps they can be discussed—although asking someone to stop leaving the top off the toothpaste after thirty years might not get you far. Some habits and personality traits can't be changed—research, however, shows people do evolve, and many things can be improved if you encourage without nagging. You have to accept your partner should do the same to you … and all people come with traits you might perceive as faults. Not expecting too much is a hard lesson, but it can be the making of your marriage, even after many years.

Long-term prospects of roses around the door at 80? Do you like that person? Do you want to share most of your time with them? Do you have enough in common? Do you like your life with that person? If mostly yes, then stay with it. sixty percent of people who get divorced later say they regret it. A marriage that has lasted 20, 25, 30 years is worth fighting for.

If not, there is no disgrace in splitting up/divorcing/separating, or of living next door to each other and being friends. People find their own ways; there are no clear-cut rules.

family

Disagreements between couples over how to treat the children can do as much serious harm to a marriage during midlife as they can when the children are very small. And conflict between parents and children, as well as you and your own parents, can also disrupt the household—or at least your peace of mind.

Now couples are having their children later—in their mid-to-late thirties is quite commonplace—this means the 50s, which were once the decade for peace, prosperity, and selfish pleasures, are the most manic of all our lives. Teenagers on the loose! Moods! Drugs! Mess! Transportation disagreements! Noise! Sex! Love angst! And then it's university problems, money worries, more drugs, alcohol, more love angst, malnutrition … Why did you have them? Why do you put up with it? Because you love them.

The trick with teens still at home is to have a strong belief that this will pass, for it will. They will, sooner rather than later in most cases, turn into lovely—or at least passable—human beings. The second trick is not to let them ruin your relationship with your partner. "Divide and rule" is their motto—don't let it happen. Single parents have the advantage here. Couples need to talk to each other about their children before they talk to the children. That way, if one of you disagrees on a course of action you work it out before the child realizes they might be able to milk the situation.

The third motto is to get and/or keep a life of your own. The one thing teens and early 20s hate more than anything is to have to feel responsible, guilty, or worried about you—they have enough trouble worrying about themselves. If you can be seen to be being happy and enjoying life, they will like that. But don't overdo it—they also want you to be there when it is important.

Forget sending them food parcels twice a week or worrying about their laundry—that is their problem. But you need to give the impression you are somewhere in the background, caring about them and hoping they are happy. Laid-back love, something like that. They also need to know they can come back to the family home at any time, once they have left—but not to sponge off you.

Avoid, at all costs, meddling, alienating them and their friends/lovers, competing for their affections and time, taking sides when there is more than one sibling, and being overprotective.

parents and dependants

Sometimes life doesn't seem fair. When breathing that big sigh of relief because the kids have finally left home or are at least showing signs of independence, you are faced with an elderly parent or in-law who can't cope on their own. Do you invite them into your house/convert the shed? Do you recognize caring for them as your duty or do you put them in the nearest nursing home and only visit on Sunday?

My view is that you should put your partner and children first and your parent second. That means discussing the situation with your own family and seeing what their views are and then, if possible, finding a solution is acceptable to all. Never decide that a parent or relative can come to live with you unless you are as near 100 percent sure as you can be that you will be able to stay the course. If taking them in will lead to divorce, it is not the right decision.

If it really isn't possible for the dependant to come and live with you—and, after all, many families don't have room—then assisted living or a nursing home is the obvious answer. Get an appointment with the managers of several locations to talk through all the problems and questions you have surrounding this decision, and you should make sure the dependant understands all the way along what is happening, as far as that is possible.

One last alternative is to share the care among you and your siblings (or the in-law siblings), which would mean the dependant moving home every few months or so.

Once a decision is made after careful thought and planning—don't feel guilty.

can they live with you?

- If your dependants are ill or infirm you might not be able to provide the care necessary. In that case you need to see what care and nursing help you can expect in the home, and what relief care for you will be available.

- Although you can feel sorry—and perhaps responsible—for that person, if you never got along with them all through your lives, it is unlikely that you will get on with them now.

- People who are dependent do tend to get crustier, not sweeter. This is worth bearing in mind.

- If you live with a relative, don't let them "rule the roost" by emotional blackmail or any other means. Any children left at home, as well as you and your partner, need to have a quality of life, too.

- Consider your own personality, and the commitments you already have in place. Do you have the time and energy to do this extra work?

- Don't feel angry if your partner feels he or she can't live with the relative in question—it isn't an obligation of modern marriage and you shouldn't feel aggrieved if this is the case.

- Are there any other people who have, morally, as big a responsibility towards the care of this person as you do—other brothers, sisters, etc.? If so, why are you taking it as your problem alone?

- Will there be advantages that are important to you or others in the household apart from the dependant? For example, if you all get on well it might be an even happier household; by taking in that person you might feel more comfortable with yourself, and so on.

firming up your friendships From the cradle to the grave, you need friends—and midlife is the perfect time to reassess your friendships ... affirming current ones, renewing old acquaintances, and even making new pals to see you through the next fifty years or so.

When you were little, you were never happier than when you had a "best friend" to play with. When you were a teenager, you wanted to be one of "the gang." In your 20s you probably had a few close friends and were adept at making new ones, while beginning to realize that friendships can easily fade away if you don't invest time in them. By the middle years, some of us have a wide circle of good friends, many kept since those early years. But others of us have managed to lose most of them along the years by putting work or family first.

If you're feeling now that you wish you'd invested more effort or time on developing, nurturing, and keeping friends, don't worry—it isn't too late to do something about it. No need for desperate measures—like a neighbor of mine who every Christmas gets out all her old cards and puts them up, or the work colleague who leaves messages for herself on her voice-mail at home so she won't feel depressed when she gets in.

reaffirming current friendships

Old, long-standing friends are a bit like marriage partners—we tend to take them for granted. This is fine up to a point—but you can't sustain a real friendship if you invest no effort for years. Friendships need feeding.

First write a list of your current friends. Not acquaintances from work or neighbors you say "Hi" to—proper friends. One survey I know of found the average person claims fourteen friends, but I feel this is an exaggeration—like the surveys on sex where we all claim to do it twice a night, every night at the age of 60. We don't want to admit the truth sometimes!

If you can write down several, good. It doesn't have to be fourteen Think about each, when you last contacted them, how much time you spend "interacting." If you feel you've been remiss in keeping that friendship alive, do something about it. But only do this if you really do want to keep in touch with that person.

For friendship to work at any age, the friend needs to bring something you need to the relationship. That's why having different types of friends usually works best. One for golf, one for drinking, one for going to the movies, one for gossiping, one for moaning, and, if you're married, a few communal marriage couple friends… you know the sort of

thing. If all your friends come into the same group (all golfing cronies, for instance) consider expanding your repertoire.

If at this stage you are wondering whether you are potentially popular enough to win over all these new friends, don't worry. Of course you are. Popularity is nothing more than giving people what they need. All the people you tend to like best as friends are those who make YOU feel good, either about yourself, or about life. That, or they affirm who you are and that others feel the same way as you. So, you do that for other people, and you will be perennially popular.

Having money can work against you more than having no money. If you are wealthy, don't slosh the cash around and don't boast. Nice people are sometimes intimidated by signs of affluence. And you don't want the kind of "friends" who think you will dip your hand in your pocket all the time.

renewing old friendships

Don't feel embarrassed about contacting someone you haven't seen or spoken to for years. It happens to everyone. Every single person goes through life and loses friends—we move, we get busy, we change. But something strange happens in midlife—we begin to think about the people we used to know at school, at college, at our first workplace, in our old hometown. Think about people you used to like. Chances are you will still like them, even if you have both changed outwardly.

Friendships that lapsed more recently can also sometimes be revived—it is very likely the person you contact will be delighted to be in touch again. If not—well, you've lost nothing; at least you tried. Give it a go—make contact by e-mail, card, or phone. You might still have a great deal to offer each other.

making new friends

Why do people think that as they get older they won't be able to make new friends? Or that they don't want new friends? Yes, it's wonderful to have a cache of people we've known for years, who know us inside out, but you should carry on bringing people into your life even at 90. They give you a new view on the world, and make you take a new look at yourself, too.

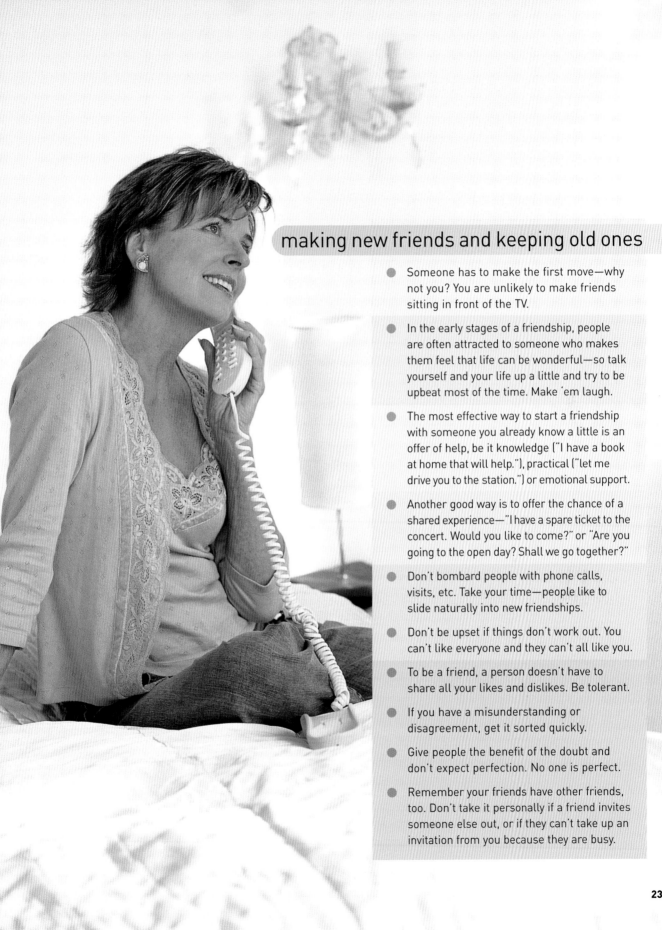

making new friends and keeping old ones

- Someone has to make the first move—why not you? You are unlikely to make friends sitting in front of the TV.

- In the early stages of a friendship, people are often attracted to someone who makes them feel that life can be wonderful—so talk yourself and your life up a little and try to be upbeat most of the time. Make 'em laugh.

- The most effective way to start a friendship with someone you already know a little is an offer of help, be it knowledge ("I have a book at home that will help."), practical ("let me drive you to the station.") or emotional support.

- Another good way is to offer the chance of a shared experience—"I have a spare ticket to the concert. Would you like to come?" or "Are you going to the open day? Shall we go together?"

- Don't bombard people with phone calls, visits, etc. Take your time—people like to slide naturally into new friendships.

- Don't be upset if things don't work out. You can't like everyone and they can't all like you.

- To be a friend, a person doesn't have to share all your likes and dislikes. Be tolerant.

- If you have a misunderstanding or disagreement, get it sorted quickly.

- Give people the benefit of the doubt and don't expect perfection. No one is perfect.

- Remember your friends have other friends, too. Don't take it personally if a friend invites someone else out, or if they can't take up an invitation from you because they are busy.

addresses and contacts

NOTE: When writing to organizations to request information, please enclose a stamped, self-addressed envelope.

SECTION 1
fuel for your new life

British Dietetic Association
5th Floor,
Charles House,
148–149 Queensway,
Birmingham B3 3HT
Tel 0121 200 8080
www.bda.uk.com

British Nutrition Foundation
52–54 High Holborn,
London WC1V 6RQ
Tel 020 7210 4850
www.nutrition.org.uk

The Food Commission
94 White Lion Street,
London N1 9PF
Tel 020 7837 2250
www.foodcomm.org.uk

Weight Watchers
Columbus Circle Station
PO Box 21053
New York, NY 10023
www.weightwatchers.com/index.aspx

Food and Nutrition Information Center
Agricultural Research Service, USDA
National Agricultural Library, Room 105
10301 Baltimore Avenue
Beltsville, MD 20705-2351
Tel: 301-504-5719
www.nal.usda.gov/fnic

SECTION 2
body for your new life

American Council on Exercise
4851 Paramount Drive
San Diego, California 92123
Tel (858) 279-8227 or 1-800-825-3636
www.acefitness.org/default.aspx

American Heart Association
National Center
7272 Greenville Avenue
Dallas, TX 75231
AHA: 1-800-AHA-USA-1
or 1-800-242-8721
www.americanheart.org/presenter.jhtml?
identifier=1200000

Exercise classes, gyms and health clubs
www.Gymuser.co.uk

National Register of Personal Trainers
0870 200 6010
www.nrpt.co.uk

Society of Teachers of the Alexander Technique
20 London House,
266 Fulham Road
London SW10 9EL
Tel 020 7284 3338
www.stat.org.uk

pilates
Body Control Pilates information line:
0870 16900000
www.bodycontrol.co.uk
www.pilatesfoundation.com

Yoga Journal
www.yogajournal.com

SECTION 3
looks for your new life

British Association of Aesthetic Plastic Surgeons
Royal College of Surgeons
33–43 Lincoln's Inn Fields,
London WC2A 3PN
Tel 020 7405 2234

American Society of Plastic Surgeons
Tel 1-888-475-2784
www.plasticsurgery.org/

Institute of Trichologists
Hairdressing and Beauty Industry
Authority
Tel 01302 380000
www.habia.org.uk

Beauty, iVillage Inc.
500 Seventh Avenue, 14th Floor
New York, NY 10018
Tel 212-600-6000
www.beauty.ivillage.com/

SECTION 4
well-being for your new life

American Psychological Association
750 First Street
NE, Washington, DC 20002-4242
Tel (800)374-2721 or (202) 336-5500
www.apa.org

Cancer Bacup
Helpline 0808 800 1234
www.cancerbacup.org.uk

American Diabetes Association
ATTN: National Call Center
1701 North Beauregard Street
Alexandria, VA 22311
Tel 1-800-DIABETES (1-800-342-2383)
www.diabetes.org/home.jsp

British Association for Counselling and Psychotherapy
1 Regent Place,
Rugby,
Warks CV21 2PJ
Tel: 0870 4435252
www.bacp.co.uk

British Association for Behavioural and Cognitive Psychotherapy
PO Box 9,
Accrington,
Lancs BB5 2GD
Tel 01254 875277

MIND (National Association for Mental Health)
Tel 0845 766 0163
www.mind.org.uk

North American Menopause Society
PO Box 94527
Cleveland, OH 44101
Tel 440/442-7550
www.menopause.org

Relate
Telephone 0845 130 4010
www.relate.co.uk

National Osteoporosis Society
Camerton,
Bath BA2 OPJ
Tel 01761 471771
www.nos.org.uk

The British Massage Therapy Council
17 Rymers Lane,
Oxford OX4 3JU
Tel 01865 774123
www.bmtc.co.uk

British Heart Foundation
14 Fitzhardinge Street,
London W1H 4DH
Tel: 020 7935 0185
www.bhf.org.uk

IBS Network
Northern General Hospital,
Sheffield S5 7AU
Tel 0114 261153

SECTION 5
time for your new life

National Mental Health Association
2001 N. Beauregard Street, 12th Floor
Alexandria, Virginia 22311
Tel (703) 684-7722
www.nmha.org/infoctr/factsheets/42.cfm

Friends Reunited
www.friendsreunited.co.uk

Match
www.match.com

Maturity Works
Tel 020 8667 0175
www.maturityworks.co.uk

Work-Life Balance Trust
www.w-lb.org.uk

Executives Recycled
Tel 08707 653821
www.executives-recycled.co.uk

Association of Retired Persons
601 E Street NW
Washington, DC 20049
Tel: 1-888-OUR-AARP (1-888-687-2277)
www.aarp.org

Saga
Saga Building,
Middelburg Street,
Folkestone, Kent CT20 1AZ
Tel 0800 414 525
01303 771 111
www.saga.co.uk

Third Age
210 Lincoln Street
Suite 302
Boston, MA 02111
www.thirdage.com

acknowledgements

All photographs © **Liz McAulay**

except the front cover © John Powell/Retna UK; pages 9, 15, 18 and 35 © Robert Harding Picture Library; and page 20 © Digital Vision.

The publisher would like to thank the following for their generosity in supplying items of clothing for photography: Next (daywear), Marks & Spencer (sportswear and underwear) and Frank Usher (evening wear).

Thanks also to the models: from CLOSE Management Ltd – Sarah Bee and her son, Francine Bloom, Suzi Conway and Janie Simmonds – and at MOT Models – Mike Morrell, Greg Sherriff, Tiffany Suchard and Joanna Woodley. And to the make-up artists: from Joy Goodman – James McMahon and Dottie Monaghan.

The author would like to express her thanks to the following people for their invaluable input and help in making this book possible: Lewis Esson, Mary Evans, Jane Turnbull, Jane O'Shea and all the rest of the team at Quadrille.

index